GN00836050

Leon Chaitow is an osteopat
Lecturer at the University of   ......ster, London, and
an internationally recognized authority on complementary
health topics. He has written over sixty books on a variety
of health-related themes and lectures widely in the UK,
US, Europe and Australia.

'Health Essentials' series

There is a growing number of people who find themselves attracted to holistic or alternative therapies and natural approaches to maintaining optimum health and vitality. The 'Health Essentials' series will help the newcomer by presenting high-quality introductions to all the main complementary health subjects. Each book presents all the essential information on a particular therapy, explaining what it is, how it works and what it can do for the reader. Advice is also given, where possible, on how to begin using the therapy at home, together with comprehensive lists of courses and classes available worldwide.

The 'Health Essentials' series titles are all written by practising experts in their fields. Exceptionally clear and concise, each text is supported by attractive and helpful illustrations.

Books in the series:

Acupuncture, Peter Mole
Chinese Medicine, Tom Williams
Hydrotherapy, Leon Chaitow
Self-Hypnosis, Elaine Sheehan

Health Essentials

HYDROTHERAPY

Water therapy
for health and beauty

LEON CHAITOW

© Vega 2002
Text © Leon Chaitow 1999, 2002

All rights reserved. No part of this book may be reproduced, stored
in a retrieval system or transmitted in any form or by any means,
electronic, mechanical, photocopying, recording or otherwise,
without the prior permission in writing of the copyright owners

ISBN 1-84333-382-1

A catalogue record for this book is available
from the British Library

First published in 2002 by
Vega
64 Brewery Road
London, N7 9NT

A member of **Chrysalis** Books plc

Visit our website at www.chrysalisbooks.co.uk

Printed in Great Britain
by CPD, Wales

Note from the Publisher:
Any information given in any book in the 'Health Essentials' series is not
intended to be taken as a replacement for medical advice. Any person
with a condition requiring medical attention should consult a qualified
medical practitioner or suitable therapist

Contents

Illustrations

1

What is Hydrotherapy?

Quite simply, hydrotherapy uses water to achieve therapeutic benefits. Water has particular properties which are unique (*see* chapter 3) and these are exploited to achieve a range of responses from the body which can relieve symptoms and improve the way the body works.

Water can be used in a number of ways: it can be applied to areas of the body; the body or parts of it can be immersed in water; various additives (such as essential oils, clay and Epsom salts) can be used in water to alter its effects; or water (especially sea water – *see* chapter 6) can be used for its buoyancy properties to facilitate exercise and movement.

Water can be used hot, warm, neutral (body temperature), cold, or as ice or even steam. Water can be applied at an even temperature (directly or via a material such as a cotton towel) and then alternated with either hotter or colder water in order to stimulate a response from the body; it can be used to 'challenge' the body to deal only with a cold application either locally or involving the whole body; or heat can be used for its relaxing and pain-relieving influences. Some methods involve a 'whole body', constitutional, response, while others target local areas (such as painful joints).

There are so many possible uses of hydrotherapy, and so much good research to validate it, that it is amazing that it is not used more widely, especially since it is cheap, efficient and enjoyable, and ideal for safe home application.

MODERN RESEARCH AND WATER THERAPY

Many people find the whole idea of using water to prevent or treat ill health quaint and slightly ridiculous. The examples of modern research which has proven the value of hydrotherapy given in this and later chapters should convince you that this is just not so. Whether used to prevent the common cold, improve fertility, 'cure' chronic fatigue, enhance immune function, help heart and circulation function or promote the healing of extremely painful lesions, hydrotherapy has within the last few years been shown to be effective, without side effects and with hardly any cost.

This is 'low-tech' medicine – it relies on very specific responses from the body to the precise application of hydrotherapy, based on a predictable pattern established over the hundreds of years of observation of how water does what it does to the body, and of how the body responds to it. Modern hydrotherapy is folk medicine brought up to date and much of it is suitable for home use for first aid, for general relief of many symptoms, and above all for improvement of well-being.

The examples of treatment using hydrotherapy discussed later are so dramatically effective, so simple to apply, and so safe, that there is nothing to stop you from copying the methods given unless you have a certain medical condition, such as heart disease or high blood pressure, or any chronic illness requiring medication.

Hydrotherapy also provides other benefits such as greater energy, improved skin function and appearance, and of course our primary objective – better health. A simple, dramatic example involves the basic process of taking a regular shower, but using colder water than usual, and in so doing cutting down the number and length of colds by half!

Preventing the Common Cold

In 1990 the Hanover Medical School decided to re-examine some of pioneer hydrotherapist Father Sebastian Kneipp's methods (*see* chapter 2), which he maintained would help to prevent infection. If the old priest's claims were accurate this would mean that the body's defence system, its immune function, could in some way be made more efficient by the use of methods devised over a century earlier, using simple water treatments as described in his book *My Water Cure*, published in English in 1899.

Fifty medical students volunteered to take part in the six-month trial. Twenty-five of them followed the old Kneipp method of taking an early morning shower which, over a period of weeks, was made increasingly colder, until after about three weeks the students were taking a two- or three-minute cold shower each day. The cold shower was stopped when they actually had a cold, and for a week afterwards. The remaining 25 students took a warm early morning shower throughout the study period.

Over the first three months there was very little difference between the two groups in the numbers of colds recorded or in their intensity and duration. But for the second three months of the trial the students taking cold showers had *half* the number of colds that the 'warm-shower' group had. And not only did the cold-shower students have fewer colds, but those that they did have were shorter (less than half as long) and far less acute.

Father Kneipp had suggested over 100 years ago that regular cold showers would have a 'hardening' effect that would protect the person from infection. He was right.[1] If regular cold showers lasting just a few minutes can have this effect, it is reasonable to ask what cold baths would do, especially when they last for closer to half an hour. This research was conducted in the early 1990s in a major teaching hospital in London, with quite remarkable results.

Thermo-Regulatory Hydrotherapy
(incremental exposure to cold baths)

The results of this important hydrotherapy research, involving 100 volunteers, were published in a four-page spread by *The European* on 22 April 1993. The Thrombosis Research Institute, at London's Brompton Hospital, which conducted the research, claims that the results prove without question the dramatic value of carefully graduated cold baths, and the next stage of the research, involving many hundreds of volunteers, is now well underway.

The method used in this research programme is called Thermo-Regulatory Hydrotherapy (TRH). The results showed that when applied correctly *(see* guidelines for home use in chapter 7) the effects of TRH included:

- A boost to sex hormone production, which helps regulate both potency in men and fertility in women.
- Renewed energy. Sufferers from chronic fatigue syndrome (ME) were found to improve dramatically: one person confined to bed for 18 hours a day in a state of exhaustion experienced 'a new lease of life', and is quoted as saying, 'From the first day I have regularly undertaken the hydrotherapy. With each day the feeling of well-being increases to such an extent that I can hardly wait for the next morning to arrive.'
- Improved circulation in people with cold extremities, along with increased levels of specific enzymes which help circulation.
- Reduced chances of heart attack and stroke because of improved blood-clotting function.
- Increased levels of white blood cells (defenders against infection).
- Reduced levels of unpleasant menopausal symptoms.
- Some of the volunteers found that their nails became harder and their hair growth improved.

Details of TRH for home application are given in chapter 7. Additional research evidence regarding the benefits of hydrotherapy will be found in later chapters (especially chapter 4).

In the next chapter we will briefly examine the history of hydrotherapy.

2

A History of Hydrotherapy

History records many cultures, including the ancient Egyptians, Greeks and Romans, the Chinese, Indians and Japanese, and the classical civilizations of South America and Mesopotamia, as using many different forms of hydrotherapy.

In more recent times, John Floyer, a doctor in Lichfield, England, who was born in 1649 and died in 1734, wrote *A History of Hot and Cold Bathing* which, published in the last days of the 17th century, went into many editions and was translated into a number of foreign languages.

The German version is said to have had a strong influence on Johann Hahn (1696–1773), who with his family developed the basis of modern water therapy in Silesia, where just a few years later one of the giants of early water treatment, Vincent Priessnitz (1799–1852), achieved amazing results when he treated people using his version of hydrotherapy which involved only variations on the use of cold water, never hot. In their excellent history of natural healing, *The Nature Doctors*, Friedhelm Kirchfield and Wade Boyle describe a typical 'treatment day' under Priessnitz in the 1840s:

Awaken at 4am to be wrapped in numerous blankets to sweat for up to several hours then plunged briefly into a cold tub. This would be followed immediately by a brisk walk, after which a simple breakfast of bread, cold milk and fruit was served. At 10am a cold douche [shower] was taken, followed by simultaneous sitz [see p59] and foot baths. A 'plentiful but coarse' dinner would be served at 1pm. The douche was repeated at 4pm and the sitz and foot baths taken again at 7pm. A supper similar to the breakfast was then served, and the

5

patient retired at 9.30pm. During free time patients walked the Grafenberg mountain trails ... about 10 miles per day, and drank copiously of cold water from the mountain springs.

Priessnitz often decided what treatment to offer only after seeing the patient's response to a cold bath. If the skin reddened he predicted a far more rapid 'cure' than if it remained pale. He became famous and worked under government authority, teaching his methods to hundreds of doctors, despite having no medical qualifications.

Many others followed his example, including Johann Schroth (1798–1856), who combined the 'water cure' with fasting. Schroth used less drastic hydrotherapy approaches than his contemporary, Priessnitz, often employing warm moist packs. However, his dietary methods were far more stringent. Priessnitz and Schroth are seen as the pioneers of what has become naturopathic medicine.

Most notable amongst other pioneer hydrotherapists was Father Sebastian Kneipp (1821–1897), whose work lives on today in Germany where there are dozens of Kneipp Kurhause using modern techniques of hydrotherapy, where patients can stay for residential care paid for under the national health system.

Kneipp treated tens of thousands of people using hydrotherapy alongside herbal therapy, diet, exercise and general 'hygienic' treatment (fresh air, sunlight, rest), and established the basis for the evolution of the modern health spa, where all these treatments would be available for the tired and stressed. He called his method 'nature cure', and strongly influenced physicians who carried his ideas to the USA in the late 19th century.

From the mid-19th century up until the Second World War a great many other, mainly German, physicians adopted hydrotherapy as the mainstay of their treatment and rehabilitation regimes, including:

- Adolph Just (1859–1936), whose own health was recovered by use of hydrotherapy and diet, and who published the landmark book *Return to Nature*. As a result of his own experience he established a sanitarium in the Hartz mountains.
- Emanuel Felke (1856–1926) who used the same methods, diet, herbs, water treatment and homeopathy, in a residential setting where stress reduction and a 'return to nature' was made possible. His Jungborn clinic also utilized loam, which has its

echoes in the 'Moor bath' and clay methods discussed in later chapters (*see* chapter 8).

- Franz Schonenberger (1865–1933) who introduced these 'natural' methods into the purpose-built Priessnitz Hospital near Berlin, Germany, in 1927.

In the UK great hydrotherapy centres such as those at Bath were developed, and similar establishments mushroomed throughout Europe, most notably in Germany, Austria, Hungary and Czechoslovakia, and later in France.

Followers of Priessnitz, and later of Kneipp, such as Benedict Lust (1872–1945), travelled to the Americas, where they enthusiastically applied the methods that these pioneers had developed. Lust introduced Kneipp's work to the USA and helped to develop what has become naturopathic medicine. By the latter part of the 20th century there were major teaching establishments in the USA (such as Bastyr University in Seattle, and the National College of Naturopathic Medicine in Portland, Oregon) where these traditional methods were taught, in highly scientific settings, to prospective doctors of naturopathy, as well as being practised in their clinics.

Earlier in the 20th century the most famous of all American spas (and in its time one of the largest in the world, with over 1,000 patients in residence at any given time) was that which grew around Dr John Harvey Kellogg (1852–1943) at Battle Creek, Michigan. Dr Kellogg is famous for the cornflake breakfast he invented in an attempt to wean his patients away from the high-fat breakfast eaten in the USA in the late 19th century. His book *Rational Hydrotherapy* was first published in 1901, and is still regarded as the best textbook ever written on the subject.

Other American innovators followed the European methods and some developed their own variations, most notably Otis G Carroll (1879–1962) who developed constitutional hydrotherapy, an almost universally applicable form of hydrotherapy treatment. It has no particular focus but seems to improve all systems and functions of the body if applied regularly (three to five times weekly). (*See* chapter 7 for details of home application.)

In the UK modern spa hydrotherapy is used as one of the centrepiece treatments, alongside fasting and dieting, manipulative methods such as osteopathy and massage, exercise, relaxation, fresh air and sunbathing. Stanley Lief (1892–1963) set the UK pattern for such establishments at Champneys, still the flagship of luxury spa treatment. Lief founded the British College of Naturopathy and Osteopathy in London (from which the author graduated in 1960) which now runs both undergraduate and postgraduate courses (to MSc level) in naturopathic and osteopathic medicine. The courses include instruction in hydrotherapy (and its clinical uses), keeping the traditions which started almost two centuries ago in Eastern Germany very much alive. One of Britain's most respected naturopathic clinics, Tyringham near Newport Pagnell, has also maintained a strong focus on hydrotherapy, and includes both American approaches (constitutional hydrotherapy), and traditional methods, as well as some innovative ideas of its own.

Best selling author Jane Alexander describes a typical day at Tyringham:
- Aqua-aerobics (pool exercise) (*see* chapter 6)
- 'Scottish douche' ('Standing naked in a shower a nurse directed a hot jet of water up and down my spine, followed by a freezing cold stream. She alternated hot and cold for several minutes before rubbing down my back with salt and allowing me to shower off ... it certainly sweeps away the cobwebs ... and apparently stimulates circulation and improves immune functioning'
  - Steam bath (seated in a sealed 'pod', with only the head free of steam, for 20 minutes)
  - Seaweed bath
  - Mud bath (*see* chapter 8)
  - Alternating hot and cold baths (*see* chapter 7)
  - Constitutional hydrotherapy ('Tyringham prescribes this procedure for anything from infertility to PMS, and from hypertension to haemorrhoids') – *see* chapter 7

In conclusion, the methods described in this book have come to us via the pioneer work of Austrian, Silesian, German, French, American and British practitioners in the field of hydrotherapy. It is an honourable tradition which has been much researched in recent years with suitably impressive results; you can read about some of these in the next chapter.

3

How Hydrotherapy Works

AMAZING FACTS ABOUT WATER

If scientists were asked to invent a substance:

- in which many other substances can dissolve (more things can dissolve in water than in any other liquid, making it ideal for transporting substances such as minerals to the body surface)
- which is almost universally available and inexpensive
- which is non-toxic and non-irritating
- which rapidly absorbs and holds a good deal of heat yet gives it up easily without cooling too rapidly
- which can store energy and turn from liquid to vapour or to a solid, while being useful in all three states

they would undoubtedly smile, scratch their heads and say, 'Why invent it? We already have it – it's called water.' Remember – at least 70 per cent of your body is water.

Water has the following major qualities, all of which we can use in hydrotherapy:

- Water is the most abundant compound (combination of elements – in this case hydrogen [about 90 per cent] and oxygen [just over 10 per cent]) on the planet.
- Water is extremely malleable; it can be made to touch almost every part of the surface of the body (and inside as well). And when absorbed in a towel or other material it can be moulded to all the contours and outer surfaces of the body to interact with the skin in remarkable ways. This makes it wonderfully useful for self-treatment.

- Water absorbs and gives out large amounts of heat, without changing its own temperature very much.

How water works on the body:

- When you apply anything *warm or hot* to tissues the muscles relax and blood vessels open more widely. This causes more blood to reach those tissues. Unless this is followed by some activity (such as the muscles contracting and relaxing during exercise) or a cold application of some sort, the tissues may then become congested which is not helpful. For this reason a cold application almost always follows a hot one in hydrotherapy methods.
- When a *short cold* application is used it contracts the local blood vessels. This has the effect of decongesting tissues, and is rapidly followed by a reaction in which blood vessels open and tissues are flushed with fresh, oxygen-rich blood.
- *Alternate hot and cold* applications produce circulatory interchange and improved drainage and oxygen supply to the tissues, whether these be muscles, skin or organs.
- Two important rules of hydrotherapy are that there should almost always be a short cold application, or immersion, after a hot one, and preferably also before it (unless otherwise stated), and that when heat is applied it should always be bearable, and never hot enough to scald the skin.

The general principles of hot and cold applications are that:

- Short cold applications stimulate circulation
- Long cold applications (more than a minute) depress circulation and metabolism
- Long hot applications leave the area congested and static and demand a cold application to help restore normality
- Short hot applications (less than five minutes) stimulate circulation, but long hot applications (more than five minutes) depress both circulation and metabolism drastically
- Short hot followed by short cold applications cause alternation of circulation, followed by a return to normal
- Hot is defined as 98–104°F or 36.7–40°C. *Anything hotter than this is undesirable and dangerous.*
- Neutral applications, or baths, at body heat are very soothing and relaxing.
- Cold is defined as 55–65°F or 12.7–18.3°C.

- Anything colder is very cold, and anything warmer is cool (66–80°F or 18.5–26.5°C) or tepid (81–92°F or 26.5–33.3°C) or neutral/warm (93–97°F or 33.8–36.1°C).

REFLEX EFFECTS OF WATER THERAPY

Certain parts of the body, when heated or cooled, will have reflex effects on the circulation of distant areas. The main reflex connections are as follows:

- The skin of feet and hands is reflexively connected with the circulation to the head, chest and pelvic regions (especially the bladder and reproductive organs, including the prostate in men).
- The skin of the lower breast bone is reflexively connected to the kidneys.
- The skin of the face is reflexively connected with the blood vessels of the head.
- The skin at the base of the neck area is reflexively connected with the mucous membranes of the nose (which is why something cold put on the back of the neck stops a nose-bleed).
- The skin overlying various spinal regions connects with the internal organs supplied by nerves from that spinal level (the lungs and heart with the upper spine; the stomach and liver with the middle spine; the bowels and abdominal organs with the lower back).
- The skin of the thighs, lower back and buttocks reflexively connects to the genito-urinary organs.
- The skin of the lower inner thighs connects with the prostate and uterus.

These reflex areas have various uses in hydrotherapy. For example, if you have a headache caused by cerebral congestion (too much blood in the head), a long cold application of more than one minute to the skin of the scalp would have the effect of constricting and therefore decongesting the vessels of the skull if the circulation could easily drain from the area; it might be impeded by muscular tension, which could be eased by gentle massage or relaxation. Other choices for congestive headaches would include:

- Alternate hot and cold applications to the head
- Cold application to the head and hot application to the feet

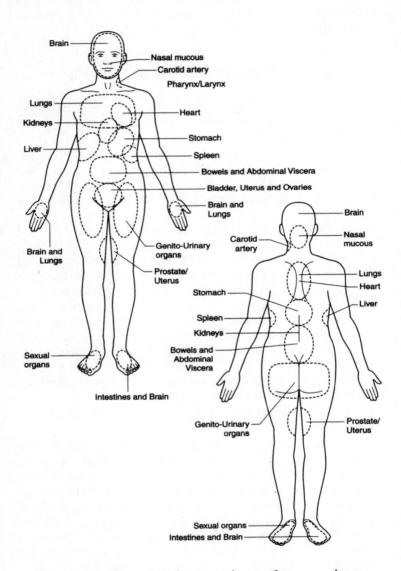

Figure 1 Skin areas reflexively connected to specific organs and parts.

- Ice pack to the throat area to reduce circulation to the head
- Cold application to the palms of the hands to reflexively decongest the head.

More of the amazing qualities of water will become apparent as the various applications are explained in the following pages. Some of the benefits come directly from the qualities of water itself, while others emanate from the substances that you can add to it. Water is a powerful ally in the quest for health and beauty.

4

What Hydrotherapy Can Do for You

Glowing good health makes you feel good and look good. And looking good – with bright eyes, soft and smooth skin, firm and flexible muscles – relates directly to being well and healthy.

Whether your aim is to maintain a sense of healthy, energetic well-being, with all its outer and inner benefits; or to restore or retain a highly efficient immune function, defending you against infection and toxicity; or to work towards regaining that ideal state of positive health – some degree of effort is called for. But it does not have to be burdensome or unpleasant. It can and should be enjoyable and fun – something that becomes an integral part of your everyday life.

Few would deny that we live in a period of constant and increasing environmental and social stress, and our state of health (whether holding on to it or getting it back) depends on how well we handle the multiple physical and emotional stresses we face. Where we can't avoid negative factors, such as pollution in the atmosphere or having to live or work in situations that promote tension, it makes sense to think about what we can do to defend our bodies and minds efficiently and, wherever possible, in ways that are pleasant. Water therapy is a highly effective and enjoyable way to achieve optimum health of mind and body.

Hydrotherapy alone is obviously not capable of solving all our health problems. It does, however, help us to retain or regain health, vitality, well-being and zest for life. It can also induce relaxation and ease pain.

There are two major areas of emphasis in health issues: keeping healthy, and getting back to a healthy state after illness. *Real* health can only be achieved when *all* your needs (biochemical, structural, emotional, spiritual) are met, and this calls for attention to diet, exercise, sleep levels and stress reduction.

HELP YOURSELF TO HEALTH

Think about when you last felt really well, full of energy, without a care or an ache or a health problem of any sort, when you could sleep easily and deeply, and wake refreshed and ready for anything. That desirable state of affairs can only exist when you are well nourished, emotionally balanced, getting enough exercise and providing yourself (or being provided) with the many and varied requirements for health.

When, for whatever reason, you slip from that balanced state, there is only one way back to health, and that is by means of the self-healing mechanisms that we all possess. Cuts heal, breaks mend, infections pass – usually without help – if your defence mechanisms are working well. Whatever treatment helps you along the way does just that – it helps you, it doesn't 'cure' you. *You* cure you.

By using hydrotherapy you can help yourself towards a better state of health. So, if pleasant water-based treatments can be combined with other health-promoting methods – such as relaxation, exercise, massage, a balanced, nutritious and delicious diet – you have a potent recipe for increased good health. We can all enjoy the benefits of traditional hydrotherapy and its modern versions, especially when the essential oils of plants and other safe, health-promoting, natural substances are added to the water used.

CONDITIONS THAT CAN BE HELPED BY WATER THERAPY

There follows a list of conditions which may benefit from the hydrotherapy methods described later in the book. This list is partial – many more afflictions can be helped by water therapy.

Anxiety

- Constitutional hydrotherapy
- Neutral bath

Hydrotherapy

- Stage two of wet-sheet pack (*see* p49)
- Various essential oil baths

Arthritis

- Constitutional hydrotherapy
- Heating compress
- Fomentations
- Full sheet pack (all four stages)
- Various essential oil baths
- Epsom salts bath
- Ice pack (if the condition is actively inflamed)
- Alternating sitz baths

Backache

- Constitutional hydrotherapy
- Fomentations
- Hot sitz bath
- Heating compress
- Full sheet pack (all four stages)
- Various essential oil baths
- Epsom salts bath
- Alternating sitz baths when the back is not in an acute phase

Bites & stings

- Ice packs
- Various essential oil applications/baths

Breathing problems

- Constitutional hydrotherapy
- Various essential oil baths
- Steam inhalations
- Heating compress (trunk and chest)

Bursitis

- Constitutional hydrotherapy
- Ice pack

16

- Alternating hot and cold applications
- Alternating sitz baths

Cellulite

- Various essential oil baths
- Local hot and cold applications

Chest (*tight, congested*)

- Constitutional hydrotherapy
- Heating compress
- Neutral bath
- Steam inhalations
- Alternating sitz baths
- Epsom salts bath (if vitality is good)
- Various essential oil baths

Chest pain (*such as intercostal neuralgia*)

- Constitutional hydrotherapy
- Fomentations
- Heating compress
- Full sheet pack (all stages)
- Neutral bath

Congestion (*local*)

If chronic choose from:

- Constitutional hydrotherapy
- Heating compress
- Fomentations
- Full sheet pack (all stages)
- Alternating sitz baths

If acute choose from:

- Ice packs or ice massage
- Local alternating compresses/applications
- Full sheet pack (first two stages only)

Hydrotherapy

Constipation

- Hot sitz bath for atonic constipation
- Full sheet pack to include stage three for bowel discomfort related to constipation

Cystitis

- Neutral sitz bath
- Various essential oil baths

Depression

- Constitutional hydrotherapy
- Various essential oil baths
- Full sheet pack (first two stages)

Detox

- Constitutional hydrotherapy
- Epsom salts bath
- Full sheet pack (all stages)
- Various essential oil baths
- Heating compress (on trunk to cover liver area)

Digestive problems

- Various essential oil baths
- Full sheet pack (first three stages)
- Heating compress

Dysmenorrhoea (painful periods)

- Various essential oil baths
- Hot sitz bath
- Fomentations

Exhaustion (fatigue)

- Alternating sitz baths
- Full sheet pack (first stage only for no more than five minutes)

- Various essential oil baths
- Cold baths as described in discussion of Thermo-Regulatory Hydrotherapy in chapter 6

Fever

- Constitutional hydrotherapy

If vitality is good:

- Full sheet pack (first stage only for five minutes or less)

To hasten the onset of a fever which is building slowly (if vitality is fair)

- Full sheet pack (all stages)
- Steam inhalations if fever is accompanied by congestion
- Epsom salts bath if sweating is needed (five minutes only)
- Heating compress (on trunk) overnight

Fluid retention

- Constitutional hydrotherapy
- Neutral bath (as long an immersion as possible)
- Full sheet pack (all stages or end after second stage if vitality poor)
- Various essential oil baths (those with diuretic effect – *see* chapter 8)
- Epsom salts bath

Haemorrhoids

- Alternating sitz baths
- Ice pack if acute
- Alternating local applications
- Hot sitz bath if constipated (use cold application to haemorrhoids after bowels move)

Headache

- Constitutional hydrotherapy

Before it is fully established:

- Mustard foot bath

Hydrotherapy

Once established:

- Essential oil baths
- Ice pack
- Full sheet pack (all stages)

If tension headache

- Neutral bath

Toxic headache

- Epsom salts bath

Heart tonic

- Neutral bath
- Full sheet pack (to include stage two)
- Cold bathing according to guidelines given in chapter 6 (if there is a heart condition for which treatment is being given, check with your doctor first)

Inflammation

- Constitutional hydrotherapy
- Alternate sitz baths
- Ice pack or ice massage
- Heating compress

Injuries

- Constitutional hydrotherapy
- Heating compress
- Ice pack
- Ice massage
- Alternating sitz baths
- Alternating hot and cold applications

Insomnia

- Constitutional hydrotherapy
- Various essential oil baths
- Full sheet pack (all stages)

- Neutral bath
- Epsom salts bath (if vitality is good)
- Heating compress (on abdominal and chest area)

Joint pain/swelling

- Constitutional hydrotherapy
- Ice pack (when acute)
- Heating compress
- Full sheet pack (all stages, especially if pain is chronic or very acute)
- Various essential oil baths
- Epsom salts bath
- Alternating sitz baths

Mastitis

- Heating compress
- Full sheet pack
- Alternating sitz baths

Menopausal problems

- Constitutional hydrotherapy
- Various essential oil baths
- Full sheet pack (all stages)
- Neutral bath
- Thermo-Regulatory Hydrotherapy bathing according to guidelines given in chapter 6

Muscle aches and spasm

- Constitutional hydrotherapy
- Fomentations
- Full sheet pack (all stages)
- Neutral bath
- Various essential oil baths
- Hot sitz bath
- Ice pack or ice massage if acute

Hydrotherapy

Pain, acute or chronic

- Constitutional hydrotherapy
- Full sheet pack (all stages)
- Neutral bath
- Heating compress to local area
- Epsom salts bath (if chronic)

Pelvic inflammatory problems

- Constitutional hydrotherapy
- Neutral sitz bath if acute
- Alternating sitz baths if chronic
- Fomentations
- Heating compress

Sinus

- Steam inhalations
- Mustard foot bath
- Alternating sitz baths

Skin sensitivity and problems

- Oatmeal bath
- Fomentations
- Full sheet pack (first two stages)
- Various essential oil baths
- Steam treatments for cleansing

Sore throat

- Constitutional hydrotherapy
- Heating compress (on throat and trunk simultaneously – two separate compresses at the same time)
- Steam inhalations to decongest
- Alternating sitz baths

Sprains

- Alternating applications
- Ice massage
- Ice pack

Stress-related tension

- Constitutional hydrotherapy
- Various essential oil baths
- Neutral bath
- Full sheet pack (all stages or end after stage two)

Toothache

- Ice pack

Varicose veins

- Alternating sitz baths

For further examples of hydrotherapy efficacy, *see* chapter 1.

Helping Kidneys and Heart

Doctors at the Royal Infirmary in Bristol tested a traditional spa treatment of full body immersion for people with fluid retention, possibly due to kidney or heart disease. The volunteers for the trial had no such problems; the doctors simply wanted to test the effects of the immersion on kidney and heart function.

The water used was that of the famous Bath spa, and the volunteers were placed in a seated position with water up to and covering their collar bones. The temperature of the water was neutral, not hot or cold to the touch, but close to body temperature. They stayed immersed for two hours, during which time blood and other samples were taken.

The results were as follows:

- Kidney function improved dramatically without any stress to the organ.
- The average weight loss due to fluid loss through urination after the immersion was over half a kilo – more than the weight of water consumed before and after the immersion.
- Sodium and potassium excretion increased markedly as a result of the immersion.
- The blood became increasingly less viscous during the first half-hour of immersion, a beneficial effect for people prone to clotting.

- The 'cardiac index' – how efficient the heart is in its pumping – was increased by a 'highly significant degree'. In other words, the heart was able to pump more effectively when the body was immersed in water. It pumped 4.6 litres a minute outside the water, increasing to 7.4 litres a minute when immersed, with *no* increase in pulse rate or blood pressure. This means that the heart pumped more efficiently *without strain*, probably because any resistance to it (the tension in the muscles and blood vessels, for example) was reduced by the pressure of the water.

When the doctors repeated the tests using tap water, the results were the same.

This test proved that the heart and kidneys can be safely helped by lying or sitting in water of body temperature (hot or cold water produces a different effect) for an hour or more. When this simple method is used to treat people with kidney and heart problems a dramatic release of retained fluid is experienced *without stress to the weak or sick organs.*

Fluid Retention Due To Liver Failure

In 1987 at the Bristol Royal Infirmary a 42-year-old male patient was treated for advanced cirrhosis of the liver using hydrotherapy. His condition had produced ascites (a huge swelling of the abdomen caused by fluid retention). The remarkable result of the treatment was published in the *Journal of the Royal Society of Medicine*.[1]

The patient was given normal diuretic treatment for his condition and a low-salt diet, but this failed to produce any benefit over a two-week period. At that point the consultants decided to try a method that had been described in a classical text over 200 years before – immersion in water. The man, who had entered hospital weighing 84 kilos and had gained weight (fluid) despite the diuretic treatment, was seated in water up to his neck, at a temperature of 35°C (body heat) for two hours each day for six days. The results were dramatic and impressive.

Over the first few hours after the hydrotherapy immersion he lost 2 kilos in weight as his urine flow improved rapidly. With a combined use of hydrotherapy and the diuretic he was down to 76 kilos by day 19 – a loss of 8 kilos in 6 days, almost all of it fluid. By that time his ascites was gone, all swellings had vanished, and by following a low-salt diet and reducing his alcohol intake his condition stabilized.

The doctors stated: 'We suggest that the use of appropriate diuretics with water immersion is a safe and effective method of treating those people with cirrhosis with ascites who fail to respond to conventional treatment.' Two hundred years earlier a report had been published of a similar case: 'A scotchman in an ascites was cured. By his girdle which I saw fell six inches [he lost 6in around the stomach] in five days, pissing freely all the time.'[2]

NOTE: Anyone with a heart or kidney condition should consult their doctor before trying to use this approach, and should obtain (from a medical library) a copy of the report on this study, 'Observations on the effects of immersion in Bath spa water' by Dr J O'Hare (and colleagues).[3]

Healing Open Wounds

A painful and seldom discussed problem affecting many people is that of anal fissures – cracked and ulcerated wounds near the anus, which are aggravated by constipation. Treatment is usually by means of expensive suppositories, creams and ointments, and sometimes by surgery. The traditional hydrotherapy treatment is usually a warm sitz bath.

A Danish hospital decided to compare modern and traditional methods and monitored just over 100 patients over a three-year period. Patients who had developed anal fissures for the first time were given one of three treatments: Lignocaine ointment (a painkiller); Hydrocortisone ointment (an anti-inflammatory); or warm sitz baths and unprocessed bran (10g taken each morning and evening) to help their constipation. The sitz baths comprised sitting in hot water 104°F (40°C) in a bathtub or plastic bowl for 15 minutes morning and evening and wherever possible after every bowel movement.

The results? Let the doctors who did the study have the last word: 'Our findings show plainly that most patients with a first episode acute posterior anal fissure can be treated successfully with warm sitz baths combined with unprocessed bran, thus avoiding the use of anaesthetic and anti-inflammatory ointments.

These other methods are less effective, more expensive and have unpleasant side effects.'[4]

Hyperthermic Treatment for Infection

In the next chapter, which explains how hydrotherapy is used by practitioners as well as in spas and clinics, we come across evidence of another amazing potential for the treatment: how, by heating the body temperature using water, it is possible to deactivate cancer cells and many micro-organisms (viruses and bacteria) because they are heat sensitive. Hyperthermia involves using baths to raise the core temperature of the body to a level similar to that which occurs when you have a fever (it is often called 'artificial fever therapy'). It is used for particular purposes such as cancer treatment and treatment of infections, including serious ones such as Aids.

This method is *not* recommended for home use unless supervised by a competent and experienced health professional because it can be quite exhausting. Again the evidence is presented to help you to gain a respect for the possibilities which hydrotherapy offers.

5

Hydrotherapy with Practitioners

All naturopaths, most osteopaths, physiotherapists and chiropractors, and many massage therapists, will have had training in some aspects of hydrotherapy. Naturopaths often prescribe some of the methods described in later chapters for home use, and some have facilities in their practices for application of methods such as constitutional hydrotherapy (*see* chapter 7).

Practitioners working on joint and muscle problems will often use simple hydrotherapy, perhaps involving hot and cold packs, or ice applied in one way or another to painful and restricted areas, before or after other manual treatment. They will usually advise home use of simple methods as well, especially in relation to painful or swollen tissues.

HYDROTHERAPY AT A SPA OR CLINIC

Home use of water therapy is valuable and safe, but it is not quite the same as the water treatment you would receive in a health spa, where it might be combined with other appropriate treatments such as osteopathy, physiotherapy, massage, aromatherapy and reflexology, and also relaxation and exercise classes and a dietary programme specifically designed for you.

Spas usually have custom-built water-treatment facilities ranging from underwater massage to many different forms of contrast and heat baths. In spas around the world, but particularly in Germany, Switzerland, France and Austria, the range and combinations of treatments are simply mind-boggling. So what happens when you go to one?

Health Hydros and Spas

Most people go to spas to relax, 'de-stress' themselves, lose weight or recharge. They seldom go with specific health complaints, although if they do have any these will be taken into account when the treatment programme is planned.

There will be an initial consultation, usually with a medically qualified person, during which the reasons you give for wanting to stay at such a place, how long you plan to stay, your medical history and an evaluation of your present level of well-being (including blood pressure and heart function) will be collated so that a programme can be devised to meet your particular needs.

Clearly if you are only going to be there for a few days the programme will be of a general nature – perhaps a light diet plus daily treatments of massage, relaxation and breathing instruction, hydrotherapy (and in some spas osteopathy, physiotherapy, and/or acupuncture, if this is appropriate), as well as exercise classes. If a longer stay is possible – say a week or more – then the programme can be more precisely targeted to your needs and might involve specific plans such as dietary or fasting regimes plus an appropriate combination of treatments.

The atmosphere at spas is relaxed, with most people spending the days lounging around in dressing-gowns between their treatments or classes and the all-important mealtimes (however light these may be). There are usually also optional sporting or recreational activities, ranging from art, cooking or flower arranging classes to guided or individual country walks, swimming, yoga, tai chi or badminton. Most people leave spas feeling renewed – and this should be your aim when applying similar methods at home.

Hydrotherapy Clinics

In more specialized hydrotherapy clinics, mainly in Germany (where many are based on the work of Kneipp – *see* chapter 2), Eastern Europe and Russia, the treatments are more focused and precise, since most people attending them have real and sometimes serious health problems.

After several hundred years of experimentation and development the equipment used in modern hydrotherapy units is now highly technical, often computer-controlled for accuracy of temperature and method of application. Applications range from specific body parts being exposed to different temperature water at the same time, with rapid contrasts being introduced at precise time intervals, to high-pressure jets being played on particular reflex regions, and use of hyperthermic methods (*see* p32).

Many of the methods used in thalassotherapy (sea water) centres are also used in 'normal' hydrotherapy clinics. There are also many hydrotherapy units attached to clinics and hospitals which focus attention on exercising in water, rather than the actual therapeutic potentials of water of different temperatures. This form of hydrotherapy is largely aimed at rehabilitation following injury or loss of function through surgery or a stroke, and is dependent on highly skilled instruction by trained physiotherapist experts.

Sea Water Treatment

Treatment involving sea water is known as thalassotherapy, which comes from the Greek word *thalassa* meaning 'the sea'. The term 'thalassotherapy' was coined in 1867 in France to describe the many therapeutic uses of sea water, sea (beach) sand, seaweed, sea mud, and other substances derived from the sea.

Thalassotherapy includes using sea water for bathing, exercising and even drinking. Unpolluted sea water has unique anti-bacterial effects due to the minute plantlife (plankton) which keeps the sea pure. Pollution can, however, overwhelm this cleansing process and modern thalassotherapy centres undergo strict testing for contamination. Sea water can be used internally and externally in all the ways in which water therapy is used, as a means of treating a wide range of ailments or just for keeping fit.

The salt content of the world's oceans, which is thought to account for many of the benefits of thalassotherapy, is around 35g per litre, rising to 42g per litre in the Red Sea, and higher still in the Dead Sea.

Sea mud, which contains algae and seaweeds, is used in some thalassotherapy centres to treat skin and rheumatic conditions by being applied to the relevant areas of the body. Similarly, dry or wet beach sand, which contains sea residues, can be used for the application of heat, for example by covering painful joints in hot sand.

A variation of thalassotherapy is 'climatotherapy', which involves use of the unique qualities of the air and climate, for example on the north-west coasts of Denmark and Germany. At such clinics sea-water aerosols are sometimes used to help breathing problems. Similarly, the prevailing sea breezes, which carry sea spray and a high level of health-promoting negative ionization particles, are used to assist inhalation.

Modern sea-water treatment centres are custom-built with complex pools of varying depth for different uses and with various temperatures of water, horizontal and vertical showers, exercise pools, 'walking pools', special foot and arm bathing areas, and 'mud bath' rooms, rest and drying rooms.

Most of these centres follow strict hygiene standards, especially in Germany and France, with the water usually being drawn from a safe distance out from the shore, and at a depth guaranteeing purity. The salt content and radioactivity is monitored and a safe bacterial count maintained. In addition, a variety of tests and precautions are followed, for example in deciding how many patients can comfortably attend the facility at any one time. The pipes used are ceramic to avoid metallic contamination, and in France no factories are allowed within 10km of thalassotherapy centres.

Conditions that thalassotherapy can treat

Skin, circulatory, rheumatic and breathing conditions, and fluid retention, are the most common problems treated at thalassotherapy facilities.

Many of the treatments involve using heat from water, mud or sand, or alternating hot and cold applications of these, which are helpful in treating various forms of arthritis. Joint stiffness and injury are improved as the treatment promotes circulatory changes leading to muscle relaxation. Further improvement is gained from specific thalassotherapy exercise programmes.

The content of the water and mud is varied to suit the needs of different skin conditions, for example by the addition of fresh or dried algae and seaweeds. Dead Sea resorts in Israel and Jordan focus attention on many conditions but have a proven record of helping skin conditions such as psoriasis.

Treatment at a thalassotherapy centre

Depending upon the sophistication of a thalassotherapy facility there might be complex treatment areas, or the whole activity might be confined to a simple bathroom.

In some facilities (both regular hydrotherapy spas and thalasso-therapy centres) 'walking pools' are designed so that the patient can walk into progressively deeper levels of water, always with railings for support, walking, sitting or standing for a prescribed length of time. Exercises might also be prescribed and performed in the pools, or baths may be given in heated sea or regular water, with exercises being performed either individually or in supervised classes.

Following such immersion the patient might receive a 'Scottish' douche, which consists of a high-pressure spray or jet of cold or hot, or alternating, sea (or regular) water applied for a short time to specific areas to achieve circulatory or reflex effects. After this, treatment in a specialized solarium involves com-bining exposure to sun (ultraviolet) light, infra-red (heat) rays, and possibly sea spray or vaporized sea water. Various mud or sand applications might be used on the joints.

In some centres small amounts of sea water, containing salts of the elements such as sulphur, magnesium and iodine, may be prescribed for drinking. For example, the potassium content might be used to help fluid retention problems, or the fluoride content might be used to help calcium metabolism if this is unbalanced. The water is either given diluted with fresh water, in its natural state, or with a juice for palatability. Amounts are small, one or two tablespoonsful at most to start with, half an hour before a meal, building gradually until four tablespoons are taken three times daily.

CAUTION: Almost all thalassotherapy facilities are medically run. An assessment of your full medical history would enable the accurate prescription of treatment. Consumption of sea water as described above, without stringent hygienic precautions, could be dangerous.

Probably the only absolute contra-indication against the use of the general thalassotherapy methods applies to pregnant women or those who are very frail, who might find the treatment too exhausting.

Where to find a thalassotherapy centre

Tourist information boards of European countries such as France (especially the Brittany region), Belgium, Italy, Russia/Ukraine (the Black Sea), Germany and Denmark should be able to provide lists of their major thalassotherapy centres. There are no thalassotherapy centres in the UK, although some spas use sea salt in some treatments.

Hyperthermia and Serious Illness

In recent years the use of hyperthermia, or artificial fever therapy, has evolved; literally extreme heating of the body for particular purposes such as the treatment of cancer and infections. Viruses and bacteria are heat sensitive, some more so than others, as are cancer cells. For this reason a number of different hydrotherapy methods of heating the body are used to encourage deactivation or death of viruses, bacteria and cancer cells.

In some clinics, most notably in Germany, up to eight hours of immersion in hot water (with frequent cool drinks and cool compresses on the head and neck) are used in treating cancer. This is, however, extremely exhausting for the patient, and should not be tried at home.

At Bastyr University, one of America's leading centres for the teaching of hydrotherapy, Aids patients were recently prescribed a series of 12 hyperthermia baths at 102°F (39°C) for 40 minutes, twice weekly, in concentrated batches for three weeks at a time, over the course of a year. The HIV virus is known to be heat sensitive; a number of studies have shown that if the core body temperature is raised, by staying in water at a temperature of 107°F (42°C) for 30 minutes or more, a 40 per cent reduction in virus activity is achieved.[1] The best way of accomplishing this continues to attract medical interest and there is little doubt that the method will continue to be refined for treating some forms of infection as well as for treating cancer.

CAUTION: On no account should you attempt hyperthermic treatment on yourself or a member of your family.

For more information on hyperthermia see Further Reading on p116.

6

Preparing for Hydrotherapy Treatments

CREATE YOUR OWN HEALTH SPA

A stay at a health spa is expensive. And while a fortnight, a week or even a weekend of being served delicious, cleansing and nutritious food, of being regularly massaged with aromatic oils, bathed (in various ways), exercised, relaxed and pampered would undoubtedly be good for you, and would enable you to return to the battle refreshed and in a better state of both mental and bodily health, *it might be no more useful in the long run than having your car valet-cleaned and polished instead of having it serviced.* Because even if you can afford all that these remarkable places have to offer, probably the most they can do is to provide a short-term respite from the daily onslaught of stress.

It makes a lot more sense to find a formula that can enable you to achieve these benefits *all the time*, whenever you need them, daily if necessary, and without the outlay of money that a stay at a health farm or spa or health-hydro demands. You could then give yourself the bonus of a periodic visit to a health spa to boost what you are doing for yourself – and give yourself a treat.

If you have a bathroom with hot and cold running water you already have the main ingredients of a home hydrotherapy spa. All you need apart from that is a bit of basic organization, some information (read on), some inexpensive materials, a bit of time for yourself and the determination to be well, healthy and full of zest. The rest should be fun.

A home spa is a common-sense approach which is within the reach of almost everyone. A home spa can be enjoyable and pampering as well as health promoting, and you can use it in whatever way you want to. How much effort you put into making it a full and 'holistic' experience is up to you.

Ingredients for a Home Spa

The core of a spa is the water treatments, but to be truly effective these need to be linked to a balanced, wholesome diet, periodically interspersed with detox periods, and accompanied by gentle but regular exercise (including breathing exercises), relaxation and – if at all possible – massage. Your home spa will then be set up for health promotion and energy gains, first aid, and treatment of specific health problems.

We are all individuals with unique characteristics and needs, and if you are to get the best out of your home health spa it is important that you devise a pattern of home care, whether for beauty or health or both, that suits your own needs and requirements. The whole process should be fun and not a burden or it could become self-defeating and add to your stress levels. You need to give yourself time, and a personal space with special qualities.

Creating a Healing Space

Sound

Your personal health spa needs to include a variety of relaxation aids and an important one is sound. You should invest in some tapes of appropriate music and sounds, such as birdsong, forest sounds, whales singing – anything you find calming. You can also buy, or obtain from your local public library, tapes that talk you though various forms of relaxation, and some books contain 'scripts' that you can record to help you through relaxation and meditation processes. Sometimes hearing your own voice is more comforting than hearing someone else – it is a very personal matter. Although this voyage of discovery into your own inner space is one you need to take alone, it may help to have initial guidance from books and tapes.

Colour

The influence of colour on our mood is very strong indeed, and you should use appropriate colours to make your home spa as restful as possible. To some extent the choice of which colours relax or energize you will be a very personal matter. There are, however, general rules that seem to apply to all of us.

- Blue and turquoise are calm colours and are 'cooling'.
- Green tends to be neutral, and while it is said to represent balance, it can make you feel lethargic.
- Mauve and violet have spiritual and balancing influences – they are calming and peaceful.
- Red is stimulating and warming, but can be irritating and oppressive.
- Pink is often said to be extremely tranquillizing, and like mauve is associated with spirituality and calmness.
- White is the colour of purity; some people find it calming, while others are influenced negatively by white walls.
- Yellow and orange can be oppressive and irritating.
- Browns and beige colours are warm and protecting.

So choose the colours that will make your personal space as restful as possible.

Light

Full-spectrum light or sunlight is vitally nourishing to us and you should try to spend some time each day outside, if not in direct sunlight then at least exposed to light without any glass (windscreens, windows, spectacles and so on) between you and daylight. For your home spa try to get hold of full-spectrum light sources (bulbs or strip lighting) which will more or less replicate the spectrum of colours provided by the sun.

Take care over the positioning of light so that your home spa is neither too bright nor too gloomy, and so that it is welcoming and pleasant.

Air

The selective choice of plants enhances air quality and beautifies any room. This is particularly necessary in modern homes, where many chemicals are found in carpets, curtains, furnishing, insulating materials, paints, and so on. Plants such as allaomena, syndonium, philodendron and spider plants all do a marvellous job of absorbing toxic fumes.

An ionizer, which costs very little, will add the benefits of negative ionization to the air quality of your home health spa. It pumps out negative ions, which energize and stimulate us positively, and it balances the tendency in most modern homes for there to be too many positive ions, which make us feel lethargic and washed out. And of course there is no substitute for getting out into the real fresh air as often as possible – daily, if you can – for a walk, or just to sit and think.

By carefully combining plants and natural materials such as cotton, wool, silk, wood and clay with appropriate colours, sounds and light, you will create a magical place for yourself.

Making Time for Health

Relaxation

There are few things in life more important than feeling at peace with yourself and with your environment, including your relationships and your work. The fact is that we need to feel good about ourselves and those around us to function well, to feel well and to be at our best. So make sure that you give yourself some time each day to reflect, relax and unwind. This is the time for some form of relaxation or meditation. A daily 10- to 15-minute period is needed for this to positively influence your life, and a weekly massage can also be wonderfully effective in helping you to relax.

Exercise

Give yourself regular time for exercise. This should include active exercise such as walking, dancing, skipping, swimming or some form of sport, always within the levels of your current fitness status. It should also involve some stretching type exercise for a balanced approach. Twenty minutes of active exercise three times a week and ten minutes of stretching exercise daily are ideal. Exercising in water (even the bath) is described on pp104–6.

Using Your Home Spa

If you add to these the exciting possibilities that the home spa offers you, you could consider giving yourself at least a further hour or two each week! The optimum allowance per week would be:

- Relaxation: 2 hours
- Massage: 1 hour
- Active exercise: 1 hour
- Stretching exercise: 1 hour
- Home spa: 2 hours

It isn't really a question of whether you can afford the time to give yourself six or seven hours a week in which to take care of your most basic inner needs – more of whether you can afford *not* to do so! And the busier you are with work or family, the more important it is to make time to look after yourself.

Of course, if you want to devote some of that time, or additional time, to use the home spa to enhance yourself cosmetically, that will also be beneficial. There is ample evidence from medical research to show that self esteem, or how we feel about ourselves, has a strong influence on our well-being. So if your health can be helped by looking after your beauty requirements, then don't feel this is selfish or over-indulgent. You have the right to indulge yourself if you wish – to enjoy a massage, to let your cares float away in an aromatic bath, to lose yourself in deep relaxation – and to use whatever safe and effective home treatment methods you want in order to enhance and heal yourself.

What Else You'll Need

Among the other requirements for your home spa which you should start to accumulate are the following:

- Bath thermometer
- Essential oils – *see* summary of suggestions for use in chapter 9
- Liquid Moor (a peat-like substance) and mud (*see* chapter 9)
- Skin brush (natural bristle) and a loofah or bath-mitten
- Two large plastic bowls
- Non-slip bath mat
- Towels, plastic sheeting, blankets, old cotton sheeting (some of which can be cut into small squares or strips for compresses and packs)
- Shower head which can adjust to give different pressures/jets
- Epsom salts (commercial), sea salt

- Floor mat or futon or thin foam mat for floor exercises and relaxation
- Skipping rope or a rebounder (mini-trampoline)
- Bathroom scales
- Suitable spoken and sound or music tapes for relaxation and imagery, and a portable player for use in the bathroom or bedroom
- Ionizer for use in the bathroom or bedroom
- Nebulizer (to vaporize essential oils)
- Vibrator/hand massager

CAUTION: If you have a serious health condition – especially if this involves diabetes, cancer, or any other degenerative disease for which you are obliged to take regular prescribed medication – you should consult your qualified health-care provider before embarking on self-treatment involving dietary changes.

The water treatments are universally safe (if you follow the guidelines closely) *except* for a few that are contra-indicated for anyone with very high blood pressure, open skin lesions, specific allergies, or diabetes. All contra-indications will be listed in the text describing the methods.

HOW TO USE WATER THERAPY SAFELY AT HOME

Using water therapy at home gives you a range of simple and efficient ways of helping yourself to feel more energetic, to improve circulation, to tone skin and muscles, to be more relaxed, to improve sleep and generally to function more efficiently. The benefits of water therapy are far from superficial; there are also very real health bonuses, such as boosting your immune system and improving the efficiency of the heart. Water treatments are also very effective at easing aches, pains, discomfort and stiffness, and they have wonderful cosmetic qualities. There are different ways of using water therapeutically, and the different methods produce different beneficial effects.

The methods of water treatment that will be described in this and later chapters include:

- Heating compress (known in Europe as 'cold' compress)
- Fomentation (usually hot damp applications)

38

- Neutral bath (for anxiety reduction/pain relief)
- Full sheet-pack (for relaxation and detox)
- Ice pack (for calming inflammation/easing pain)
- Steam inhalations (for breathing problems/sinus congestion)
- Alternating (or single) baths, sitz baths or local immersions (for circulatory stimulation/alteration)
- Full baths of various types
- Exercising in water for numerous benefits (*see* p104 for details)
- Use of various additional substances in water – including essential oils, special mud (Dead Sea, for example) and similar substances

Among the proven effects of specific types of water therapy are:

- A reduction in general anxiety and feelings of being stressed, pressured and unable to relax. These can be helped enormously by use of a neutral bath or wet-sheet pack.
- Some methods reduce the sensitivity of nerve endings which report pain. Cold applications are good for this (using ice, for example), as are alternate hot and cold applications – wet towels can be laid on the area or, if the painful part is small, such as a hand, it can be alternately 'dunked' in contrasting water for the same effect.
- A calming of inflammation, which often accompanies pain, can be achieved using alternating methods (cold/hot/cold) or cold alone for the appropriate length of time.
- Compresses and various contrast (hot and cold) methods can reduce local swelling and congestion, such as occur with strains.
- Long cold applications, lasting more than a minute, reduce the speed of flow of blood to the area being treated, while hot applications encourage increased blood flow. By using alternations of hot and cold, circulation can be stimulated, improving skin and tissue tone and relieving the symptoms of poor circulation.
- Inactivity as well as overuse can reduce circulation to muscles and joints, leading to stiffness and sometimes pain, and this can be helped by simple methods such as contrast bathing, 'warming' compresses, cold douches, and hot and cold applications.
- Stiffness is eased when muscles relax. Hot applications can help this, as can 'warming' compresses (they are applied cold, but warm up because they are insulated) and alternating hot and cold applications or immersions.

- There are many ways of using different substances in water to assist in pain relief, including Epsom salts baths and a range of essential oils.
- Regular cold showers help reduce the incidence of colds and infection.
- Steam can be used with or without suitable aromatic herbs and oils to reduce the pain of chest and sinus congestion.
- A variety of benefits, for example involving skin conditions, can be gained by use of hydrotherapy adjuncts such as essential oils and mud or clay products (*see* chapter 9).

This and the next chapter provide some guidelines to enable you to use many of these methods safely at home and reap their benefits. It also gives some important advice about conditions in which you should *not* use water therapy.

CAUTION: There are certain situations in which water therapy should only be used with caution or not at all. For example, people with poor circulation or low vitality should not receive extreme contrasts of temperature; it is better for them to use a contrast of warm to cool rather than hot to cold applications. No one should use water therapy soon after a meal; wait for at least an hour and a half.

CAUTION: Diabetics should avoid any heat treatments to their legs.

Water therapy should *not* be used:

- On extremely fragile skin
- Where skin conditions are irritated by moisture
- Over areas of numbness
- Where there are serious circulatory conditions

– although in these instances it is worth checking with a suitable health-care professional, because treatment might be helpful but only under special instruction.

Skin Health

Your skin is not just the envelope which surrounds you – it is a powerful and vital organ. It might seem strange to consider it in this way, but your skin (when healthy) is a 'second lung' through which your body eliminates a great deal of waste material. Our circulatory system carries metabolic wastes, which are produced constantly as by-products of our normal body functions, along tiny capillaries to the skin, where they pass out through the pores.

The outer surface of the skin itself is made up of 'dead' cells which are constantly shed, but when these dead skin cells become covered with microscopically small dirt particles and oils (which you also produce yourself), the easy elimination processes of the body through the pores of the skin can be blocked or slowed, leading to blemishes, pimples and blackheads.

There are several easy ways to use water therapy to stimulate the circulation to the skin so that wastes are delivered more efficiently, and to help clear away the obstructions caused by dead skin cells and debris on the surface, so opening up the pores and enabling them to function more efficiently.

Other benefits of *regularly* treating the skin with hydrotherapy include improved tone and the mobilization of any fatty deposits lying below the skin surface (cellulite). Clearing cellulite depends on improved circulation and drainage of the tissues, and water treatments help to achieve this splendidly.

Overall health will also benefit when the skin is working efficiently, because levels of toxicity drop, thereby putting less strain on other organs of elimination such as the liver, kidneys, bowels and lungs. Minor problems such as chronic catarrh can improve or vanish, because when the skin does its job properly there is less need for other means of removing toxins, such as excretion through the mucous membranes.

Any tendency to unpleasant body odour will also improve with hydrotherapy treatments, because bacteria on the skin surface, which can cause or aggravate body odour, will have less chance to operate, and sweat deposits will be cleared away more efficiently.

Another benefit is that more energy will be available, and greater vitality, as toxic deposits are removed from the system. The final by-product of skin-focussed hydrotherapy might actually be a primary objective for many people – firmer and clearer skin, with a better colour and surface condition.

Hydrotherapy Skin Self-care

There are a few methods that can be used regularly and some that can be used now and then, selectively, when they are indicated by various conditions. Some work on the surface of the skin, while others work more deeply, stimulating circulation to and through the skin. Both are necessary to get the skin working efficiently.

While skin is a protective envelope, it also allows some passage through itself *in both directions*. So as well as eliminating wastes, it also allows nutrients and herbal essences in. By using special mixtures of nutrients and salts, as well as essential oils from plants, a profound beneficial influence on the way the body functions can be achieved.

Home hydrotherapy for skin enhancement (the methods are described later in this chapter and the next) includes:

- Treatments aimed mainly at detox and improved skin function, at least one of which should be used regularly – daily if possible
- Whole-body systematic methods, which influence circulation and general metabolism, and which should be selected from and applied once or twice a week
- Local methods of treatment

The methods that work mainly on skin function and detox include:

- Skin brushing
- Salt glow
- Moor bath
- Epsom salts bath
- Trunk pack

Those that stimulate overall circulation and improve general metabolism, as well as improving skin function, include:

- Full body pack
- Sitz baths
- Sauna
- Stimulating showers
- Aromatherapy and herbal baths

A variety of hydrotherapy methods, many of which can be applied at home, are described in the next chapter.

42

7

Home Hydrotherapy Treatments

HYDROTHERAPY FOR GENERAL HEALTH AND SYMPTOM CONTROL

The range of hydrotherapy methods described for use at home represents only a part of what might be available at a modern hydrotherapy clinic or spa. This is because these methods have been selected above all for safety, for relative ease of application, and also for their proven effectiveness.

Most act in a general way – they are not specific treatments, but methods which by helping circulation, detox and general relaxation will support the constant effort of the body to heal

---

IMPORTANT NOTES

- Choose the easiest and most convenient method of application for home use.
- Do not use more than one method on any one day.
- To get the best results, some methods (such as sitz baths, wet-sheet packs, compresses, hot/cold local-area bathing) should be repeated every day or two, for one to two weeks, especially where the condition is chronic.
- Methods such as 'constitutional hydrotherapy' and 'Thermo-Regulatory Hydrotherapy' need to be applied for some weeks or months before benefits will be noted specifically because they aim over time to modify the way the whole body functions, or the way its circulatory system operates, and this does not occur rapidly.

---

itself and to become more efficient. Some require the assistance of another person, but all are relatively simple. All the methods offer considerable benefits towards general health enhancement or symptom relief.

HYDROTHERAPY METHODS

The methods given in this chapter have been divided into:

- Applications to the body (compress, fomentation, pack and so on), some of which are applied to a part of the body, some to the whole body; some of which are single temperature, and some of which involve alternating temperatures.
- Placing the body, or part of the body, into water, sometimes at one temperature, and sometimes alternating the temperature.
- Use of methods which involve the addition of substances to the water (Epsom salts, essential oils, mud and so on).
- Adjunctive approaches, for example skin brushing and salt glow methods, ice massage and steam inhalations.

COMPRESSES, FOMENTATIONS AND PACKS

Heating Compress

This is called a 'cold compress' in Europe and is a simple but effective method. It involves the use of a piece of cold, wet material (cotton is best), well wrung out in cold water and then applied to an area which is immediately covered in a way that insulates it and allows body heat to warm the cold material. Plastic is often used to prevent the damp from spreading and to further insulate the material.

A reflex stimulus takes place when the cold material first touches the skin, leading to a flushing away of 'old' blood from the tissues, and a return to them of fresh, oxygenated blood. As the compress slowly warms there is a deeply relaxing effect and a reduction of pain.

This is an ideal method for any of the following:

- painful joints
- mastitis

44

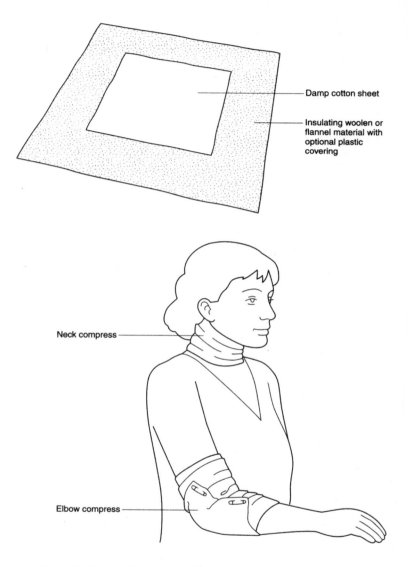

Damp cotton sheet

Insulating woolen or flannel material with optional plastic covering

Neck compress

Elbow compress

Figure 2 Heating Compresses. These are known in Europe as 'cold compresses' because they start cold and warm up.

- sore throat (the compress should be placed on the throat from ear to ear, supported over the top of the head)
- backache (ideally the compress should cover the abdomen and the back)
- sore tight chest from bronchitis

Materials

- A single or double piece of cotton sheeting large enough to cover the area to be treated (double thickness for people with good circulation and vitality, single for those with only moderate circulation and vitality)
- One thickness of woollen or flannel material (towelling will do but is not as effective) *larger* than the cotton material so that it can cover it completely
- Plastic material (the same size as the woollen material)
- Safety pins
- Cold water

Method

- Ring out the cotton material in cold water so that it is damp but not dripping wet.
- Place this over the painful area and immediately cover it with the woollen or flannel material, and the plastic material, and pin the covering snugly in place.
- The compress should be firm enough to ensure that no air can get in to cool it, but not so tight as to impede circulation.
- The cold material should rapidly warm and feel comfortable, and after several hours it should be virtually dry.
- Wash the material before reusing it as it will absorb acid wastes from the body.
- Use a warming compress up to four times daily with at least an hour between applications if it is found to be helpful for any of the conditions listed above. Ideally leave it on overnight.

CAUTION: If for any reason the compress is still cold after 10 minutes (the compress may be too wet or too loose, or the vitality may not be adequate to warm it), remove it and give the area a brisk rub with a towel.

Fomentations

The application of damp heat to an area leads to an increased circulation to that region, followed by increased metabolic activity involving the whole body, sweating, tissue relaxation and reduction in pain or spasm.

Fomentations are useful for:

- pain and congestion, especially involving muscle spasm and tension
- lumbago and neuralgia between the ribs
- dysmenorrhoea (painful periods)
- kidney stones (renal colic)

CONTRA-INDICATIONS: Do not use fomentations in all cases of cancer, heart disease, diabetes mellitus, circulatory problems of the legs, haemorrhage, or sensitive skin.

Materials

- Sheet
- Blanket
- Towels
- Very hot water
- Woollen material for fomentation (a towel will do but is less efficient)
- Bowl with hot water (and mustard if you want it to be super-efficient)
- Bowl with cold water, or access to a cold water tap
- Hot-water bottle (for method 2)

Method 1

This treatment is impossible to do for yourself so someone has to help with the applications.

- Sit in an upright chair with your feet in a bowl of bearably hot water (104°F or 40°C) in which two or three teaspoonsful of mustard powder have been dissolved.
- Uncover the area to be treated, and have the sheet and blanket handy to cover this and as much of the body as possible once the fomentation has been applied.

- Lightly wring out the woollen or towelling fomentation material in very hot water (the more water retained the more effective the fomentation) and place this immediately between several layers of dry, larger towels.
- Apply the insulated hot towels to the painful area and cover immediately with the sheet and blanket.
- If the fomentation is too hot for comfort, remove it for a few seconds, dry the skin, and then replace it.
- Change to a new fomentation application every five minutes, but between each application place a cold wet towel on the area for a few seconds.
- After the second fomentation application, or when sweating begins, apply a cold towel to the forehead.
- Repeat the applications of hot fomentations three or four times.
- After the last fomentation is removed use a damp, cold towel to friction the area, and the body as a whole, briskly (except if you are treating dysmenorrhoea) and then rest in a warm and comfortable position for half an hour to an hour.
- This treatment can be done daily if helpful, but the skin should be protected by Vaseline or something similar if it is repeated frequently.
- The heat of fomentations promotes sweating and elimination of toxic wastes. It also relaxes local spasm, thus reducing pain.

Method 2

- Lie down on an open sheet and blanket with a hot-water bottle by your feet.
- The material to be used for the fomentation should be wrung out in very hot water, placed between the insulating towels and applied to the area being treated.
- Cover with the sheet and blanket and leave for four to five minutes.
- Then remove it and apply a cold compress to the head while preparing the next fomentation.
- Repeat this process three times.
- Finish off (after the last fomentation has been removed) with a friction of the whole body using a mitten or towel.
- Wrap in the sheet and blanket and rest for at least half an hour.

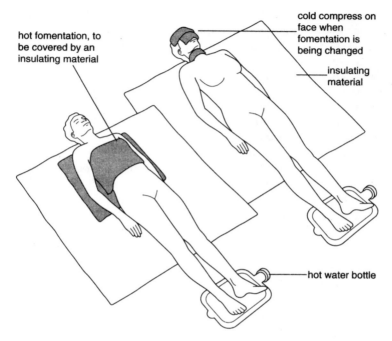

Figure 3 Fomentation (method 2)

Full Wet-Sheet Pack

The way a wet-sheet pack works depends on how it is applied. The effects of full sheet pack treatment can be remarkable in that it passes through four distinct stages of activity, each of which has different effects on the person receiving it. It is therefore useful for treating a variety of conditions.

The four stages are:

- An initial cooling stage, useful for general weakness or if there is a fever. This stage lasts no more than five minutes.
- A neutral stage, when the pack is the same temperature as the body, which has the same effects as a neutral bath, and is particularly helpful in treating agitation, anxiety and nervousness. This stage may last for half an hour or more depending upon how quickly your body heat warms the wet material.

- A hot stage, which helps in a number of health conditions but is most useful for pain problems such as sinus congestion, bowel discomfort (especially if constipated) or conditions such as colitis.
- A stage when sweating becomes profuse, which is used for general detox and to assist the elimination of the residues of drugs, including tobacco. It can also be used during some infections to hasten the fever process, but only under supervision.

CONTRA-INDICATIONS: Avoid stages 3 and 4 if you are very anaemic or very weak or debilitated. Being wrapped, mummy-like, can be claustrophobic, so there should always be someone on hand to help with removal of the pack in case this happens or if you feel unwell. Do not use this treatment if you have a skin condition that is exacerbated by water. Anyone with diabetes should take advice before using a wet-sheet pack.

Materials

- Two cotton sheets
- Two wool blankets
- Towels
- Pillow
- Hot-water bottle
- Hand towel

Method

This treatment is impossible to do for yourself, so have someone on hand to help you.

- Place a blanket on the bed, fully open.
- Have a warm shower, and without drying yourself get your helper to wrap you in a cold wet sheet, which should have been *well* wrung out in water at 60–70°F (15–21°C).
- The younger and more vital the person receiving the pack, the more water can be left in the sheet, but it should never be dripping wet when applied.

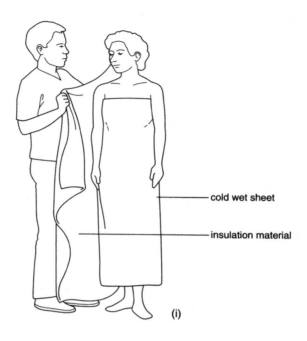

cold wet sheet

insulation material

(i)

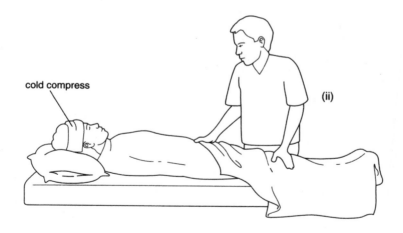

cold compress

(ii)

Figure 4 Full wet-sheet pack

51

- Working swiftly, the damp cold sheet should be wrapped from under the armpits so that it fits snugly to the body right down to the ankles, and should be immediately covered by a second, dry sheet before you lie down on the blanket Fig. 4(i). This should then be wrapped around you from neck to feet with no sheet visible (so avoiding contact with the air, which would keep it cool).
- The second blanket should be placed over the first one and fitted snugly Fig. 4(ii).
- Use towels and/or a neck pillow to insulate areas such as the neck where the blanket may not be enclosing the pack efficiently.
- Place a hot-water bottle near the feet.
- Speed of operation is essential as chilling will occur if the work is done slowly.
- When the 3rd and 4th stages (refer to description of stages given above and what conditions they are most useful for) are reached (the pack feels hot and you start to sweat), a cold compress to the forehead is a good idea, as are sips of water if you feel thirsty – sweating can be profuse in stage 4 so water replenishment is usually necessary.

The pack can be discontinued at any stage. For full benefit it should run its course, which takes up to three hours or more depending on your vitality, that is, how quickly you heat the sheet. If at any time after the first few minutes the pack is uncomfortably cold the treatment should be stopped and a brisk friction applied to the whole body surface using a mitten or dry towel to stimulate circulation. The failure of the sheet to warm up would indicate either that the sheet was too wet or the water too cold, or that the insulation was inadequately applied.

The Trunk Pack

This is a modification of the full-body wet-sheet pack, but is less difficult to apply and also less demanding on your energy – the wet-sheet pack can leave you feeling a bit limp for a day or so at first. Its objective is to stimulate elimination through the skin but also to influence circulation through the pelvic and abdominal areas.

Materials

- Large bath towel or a strip of blanket
- Strip of cotton material
- Safety pins
- Blanket

Method

Fold a thick towel in two or three, or have available a piece of blanket, wide enough to cover the area from your armpits to your navel and long enough to go right around you with some overlap. Onto this place one thickness of damp, well-wrung-out cotton material which is at least an inch narrower than the covering material and which can wrap around you once without overlap. Place these on a bed and lie on top, wrapping the material over to cover the entire area between your navel and your armpits. Quickly fold and safety-pin it, or have someone do this for you. Cover yourself with a blanket and rest.

The cold, damp cotton should warm very rapidly if it is well wrapped with no damp edges protruding, not too wet (it needs to

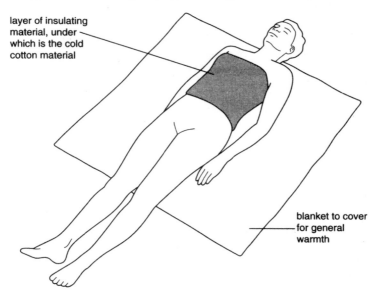

layer of insulating material, under which is the cold cotton material

blanket to cover for general warmth

Figure 5 Trunk pack

have been well wrung out) and firmly pinned. If it fails to warm within five minutes take it off, briskly friction the skin and abandon the treatment for that day. Otherwise keep the pack on for not less than an hour, and ideally for three to four hours so that it is virtually dry by the time it is taken off. The best way is to sleep with it on, but it can be done during the day if you can stay resting. The cotton must be well washed before reuse as it absorbs acidic wastes from the skin.

Alternating Hot and Cold applications: Constitutional Hydrotherapy (Home Application)

Constitutional hydrotherapy has a non-specific 'balancing' effect, reducing chronic pain, enhancing immune function and promoting healing. There are no contra-indications since the degree of temperature contrast in its application can be modified to take account of any degree of sensitivity or frailty.

Materials

- Somewhere to lie down
- Full-size sheet folded in two, or two single sheets
- Two blankets (wool if possible)
- Three bath towels (when folded in two each should reach from side to side between shoulders and hips)
- Hand towel (the same size as the large towel folded in two)
- Hot and cold water

Method

This method cannot be self-applied; help is needed.

- Undress, and lie supine between the sheets and under the blanket.
- Your helper places two hot folded bath towels (four layers) onto your trunk, covering your shoulders to your hips, side to side.
- Cover with the sheet and blanket and leave for *five minutes*.
- Return with a single layer (small) hot towel and a single layer cold towel.
- Place the 'new' hot towel on top of the four 'old' hot towels and 'flip' so that the hot towel is on the skin, and remove the old towels. Immediately place the cold towel onto the new hot

54

towel and flip again so that cold is on the skin; remove the single hot towel.

- You are covered with a sheet and left for *ten minutes* or until the cold towel is warmed.
- The previously cold, now warm towel is removed, and you turn onto your stomach.
- Steps 2 to 6 are repeated on your back.

Notes

- If using a bed protect it from getting wet.
- 'Hot' water in this context is at a temperature high enough to prevent you leaving your hand in it for more than five seconds.
- The coldest water from a running tap is adequate for the 'cold' towel. In hot summers you can add ice to the water in which this towel is rung out, if the temperature contrast is acceptable to you.
- If you feel cold after the cold towel is put in position, the helper can use back, foot or hand massage (through the blanket and towel) and/or use visualization – you can think of a sunny beach, for example.
- This is a very versatile treatment: by varying the differential between hot and cold, for example by reducing it for someone whose immune function and overall degree of vulnerability is poor, and using a large contrast, from very hot to very cold, for someone whose constitution is robust, the application is suitable for anyone.
- Apply daily, or twice daily if needed.

> NOTE: When constitutional hydrotherapy is offered at a clinic (widely available in the USA, but also at Tyringham Clinic in the UK – *see* Useful Addresses) there are additional variations to the method which cannot be included at home, often including electrotherapy applied to the back and the abdomen.

Ice pack

Ice decongests the tissues as it melts over them because of the amazing amount of heat it has to absorb to turn from solid into liquid. Ice treatment is helpful for:

- all sprains and injuries
- bursitis and other joint swellings or inflammations (unless cold aggravates the pain)
- toothache
- headache
- haemorrhoids
- bites

> CONTRA-INDICATIONS: Do not use abdominal application during acute bladder problems; over the chest with acute asthma; or if any health condition is aggravated by cold.

Materials

- Piece of flannel or wool material large enough to cover the area to be treated
- Towels
- Ice
- Safety pins
- Plastic
- Bandage

Method

- Place crushed ice onto a towel at a thickness of an inch or so, then fold and pin the towel to contain it.
- Place the wool or flannel material onto the site of the pain and put the ice pack onto this.
- Cover the pack with plastic and use the bandage to hold everything in place.
- Protect clothing and bedding with additional plastic and towels.
- Leave the pack in place for up to half an hour, and repeat after an hour if helpful.

BATHING METHODS

Neutral Bath

Placing yourself in a neutral bath, in which your body temperature is the same as that of the water, creates a profoundly relaxing

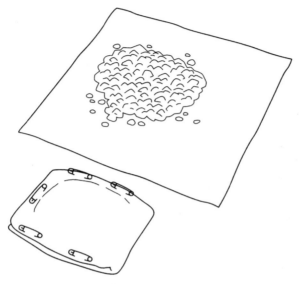

Figure 6 Ice pack

influence on the nervous system. This was the main method of calming violent and disturbed patients in mental asylums before the introduction of tranquillizers.

A neutral bath is useful in all cases of anxiety, for feelings of being stressed, and for relieving chronic pain and insomnia. It is ideal for reducing excessive fluid if retention is a problem, and is a general tonic for the heart.

CONTRA-INDICATIONS: Do not use with skin conditions which react badly to water, or if there is serious cardiac disease. In the latter case this method may help, but get professional advice first.

Materials

- Bathtub
- Water
- Bath thermometer

Method

- Run a bath as full as possible and with the water as close to 97°F (36.1°C) as possible, and certainly not exceeding that level.
- Get into the bath so that the water covers the shoulders, and support the back of the head with a towel or sponge.
- The thermometer should be in the bath to ensure that the temperature does not drop below 92°F (33.3°C).
- The water can be topped up periodically, *but must not exceed the 97°F/36.1°C limit*. The duration of the bath should be anything from 30 minutes to four hours – the longer the better for maximum relaxation.
- After the bath pat dry quickly and get into bed for at least an hour.

Alternate Bathing

By alternating hot and cold water in different ways it is possible to greatly improve circulation, and so positively influence many aspects of your health, such as an increase in energy and an improved, clearer complexion.

- Alternate bathing is useful for all conditions that involve congestion and inflammation, locally or generally, and for an overall tonic effect.
- Alternating sitz baths are ideal for varicose veins and haemorrhoids.

CONTRA-INDICATIONS: Alternate bathing should not be used if there is haemorrhage, colic and spasm, acute or serious chronic heart disease, or acute bladder and kidney infections.

Materials

- Containers suitable for holding hot and cold water
- If the whole pelvic area is to be immersed, then large plastic or other tubs (an old-fashioned hip bath is best) are required, along with a smaller container for simultaneous immersion of the feet
- Bath thermometer

- Hot and cold water
- Special ingredients, such as mustard, for some conditions

Method
- If a local area such as the arm, wrist or ankle is receiving treatment, then that part should be alternately immersed in hot and then cold water following the timings given below for alternating sitz baths.
- For local immersion treatment ice cubes can be placed in the cold water for greater contrast.
- If the area is unsuitable for treatment by immersion (a shoulder or a knee could be awkward), then application of hot and cold temperatures to those regions is possible by using towels soaked and lightly wrung out in water of the appropriate temperature, again following the same time scales as for sitz baths.

Alternating Sitz Baths

These baths involve the immersion of the pelvic area (buttocks and hips up to the navel) in water of one temperature, while the feet are placed in water of the same or a contrasting temperature. The sequence to follow is:

- 1–3 minutes seated in hot water (106–110°F or 41–43°C)
- 15–30 seconds in cold (around 60°F/15°C)
- 1–3 minutes hot
- 15 seconds cold

During the hip immersions the feet should if possible be in water of a contrasting temperature, so when the hips are in hot water, the feet should be in cold, and vice versa. If this is hard to organize, the alternating hip immersions alone should be used.

Single Temperature Bathing

These are full or partial baths where no alternation of temperatures occurs.

Hot Sitz Bath

A hot sitz bath, with no alternation of hot and cold, but simply pelvic immersion in hot water, is of proven value in helping speed the healing of painful anal fissures (*see* chapter 2), as well as haemorrhoids, dysmenorrhoea, prostate and bladder inflammation, pelvic inflammatory disease and atonic constipation.

CONTRA-INDICATIONS: Hot sitz baths should not be used by anyone with a diabetic condition.

Materials

- Containers suitable for holding hot and cold water
- If the whole pelvic area is to be immersed, then large plastic or other tubs (an old-fashioned hip bath is best) are required, along with a smaller container for immersion of the feet
- Bath thermometer
- Hot and cold water
- Special ingredients, such as mustard, for some conditions

Method

- If a hip bath is available, then sit in it in hot water (106–110°F or 41–43°C) with the feet in a separate container of water a few degrees warmer.

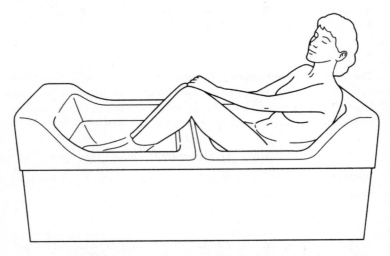

Figure 7 Sitz bath, immersing two parts of the body in water of contrasting temperatures.

- If a regular bath is used, sit in it in hot water up to the navel, knees bent so that they are out of the water, and feet immersed.
- Apply a cold towel to the forehead during the treatment. If anal fissures are being treated the time spent in the bath can be up to 30 minutes.
- For other conditions eight minutes is adequate.
- At the end of the bath rub the immersed area briefly with a towel that has been wrung out in cold water.
- If you have prostate problems, hold the damp cold towel between your legs for ten seconds or so to cool the perineal area between the rectum and the testicles.
- In some conditions, such as acute cystitis, a neutral sitz bath is useful. This involves pelvic immersion in water of the same temperature as the body for up to 30 minutes.

Full Baths

These are useful for conditions such as unnatural tiredness, anxiety, muscular stiffness, digestive problems, breathing difficulties, skin problems, menopausal symptoms, headaches, nervous complaints, cellulite and chronic painful conditions such as arthritis and rheumatism They are contra-indicated only for people whose skin is sensitive or allergic to whatever is being added to the bath (essential oils and so on).

For suggestions as to ingredients which can be added to baths refer to notes on essential oils, Moor, mud and clay bathing in chapter 8

Thermo-Regulatory Hydrotherapy (TRH)

In chapter 2 a brief description was given of the benefits of Thermo-Regulatory Hydrotherapy (TRH). There are four stages to TRH, and it is essential to 'train' the body towards the beneficial response by going through these stages in the order described. The sequence of standing, sitting and then lying in the water may not be achieved before a month or so of gradually increasing exposure to the water, and should not be rushed. The sequence described here is an average, and runs for around three months. Many people take six months to achieve the same level of exposure (length of time in the water, and degree of cold of the water)

These variables can be altered to meet individual reactions and are given as examples only. You may wish to move faster – have colder temperatures – or take longer to achieve the very cold levels. The effects will be beneficial whichever approach is taken.

Materials

- Bath
- Bath thermometer
- Watch
- Bath mat

The bathroom should be a comfortable temperature. The temperature of the water should be between 54.9°F and 65°F (12.7°C and 18.3°C) – colder for hardy people with strong vitality, and less cold for those who are more sensitive or frail. Whichever temperature is chosen start with the coldest that you can tolerate.

Stage 1

Stand in cold water in the bath for between three and five minutes as your internal thermostat (a part of the brain called the hypothalamus) starts to respond. Do not stand still, but walk up and down in the bath, or march on the spot. Be sure you have a non-slip mat in place if you try this. This process of standing in the water for three to five minutes is always a part of the process, even when after some weeks you sit in the water after standing. This is a conditioning phase and must not be skipped. For the first ten days simply walk up and down in the water for three to five minutes, and then get out of the bath. On a daily basis the water should be made just a little colder each time if possible.

Stage 2

After ten days to two weeks of the standing phase only, your internal thermostat will be primed, and following standing you should sit in cold water for another three to five minutes – up to your waist ideally – so that the pooled blood in the lower half of your body is cooled and further influences the hypothalamus. This phase of the treatment – standing for three to five minutes, followed by sitting for three to five minutes – lasts for a further two to three weeks.

Stage 3

This is the most important part of the programme, in which you need to immerse your entire body up to the neck and back of the head in cold water (after first standing and then sitting). A month or so of standing and then sitting as described has led to the point where the full bath is possible and useful, but those stages (standing and sitting) are always used at each bath before lying down.

While doing so move your arms and legs gently and slowly to ensure that the slightly warmer water touching your skin (warmed by you) is not static, so that the cooling effect continues. This stage (immersion up to the neck) lasts between 10 and 20 minutes.

Stage 4

This stage is for 'rewarming', and as this takes place a warm, glowing sensation will be felt in various precise locations such as the chest, feet and between the shoulder blades. Give yourself a brisk rub down with a towel, and then do some active exercise for a minute or two, such as running on the spot, walking up and down, rebounding or skipping.

The variables of how cold the water is and how long is spent in it allow this to be modified to a great extent, so that almost anyone, no matter how sensitive they are to cold, can slowly acclimatise to the challenge which the process offers.

If someone wants to run a marathon they start training by challenging the body to exercise a small amount, and incrementally increase the level of training until the body is ready run 25 miles. In weight training you do not start by lifting heavy weights, but challenge the muscles to lift light, and then heavier ones, until you are ready for the very heavy weights. In TRH the process of challenge if the same – with a response of better circulation and overall immune efficiency.

> CAUTION: Thermo-Regulatory Hydrotherapy is *not* recommended for anyone with well-established heart disease, high blood pressure or chronic diseases requiring regular prescription medication, unless their doctor has been consulted and has approved its use.

Jacuzzis and Hot Tubs

If you have access to a hot tub or jacuzzi this can be a help in applying heat to the painful areas of your body, and the underwater jets can apply beneficial massage as well. They are increasingly common in health clubs, health centres and better hotels, and in more and more private homes.

Many rehabilitation centres and hospitals use whirlpool baths and jacuzzis for treating pain, wounds, skin sores, chronic swellings and specific joint problems such as tennis elbow and arthritic knees. Circulation is also dramatically toned and muscles become more relaxed – and so will you – after a while in these super baths.

> NOTE: After any such hot treatment always apply a short cold treatment (such as a towel wrung out in cold water and briskly rubbed over the skin for ten seconds or so) to any painful area being treated or to the body as a whole (a short tepid shower would do) to stimulate circulation. But do not do this if you are aiming only at relaxing; just dry off, lie down and rest.

HYDROTHERAPY WITH ADDITIONAL SUBSTANCES

Simple Detox Bath

For a simple Epsom salts bath to encourage relaxation, easing of stiffness or aches and for strong detox, dissolve between 2 and 4lb (0.9 to 1.8 kilos) in the hot water and soak in this for 20 minutes. Briskly rub dry and get into a warm bed. Expect to perspire profusely.

Single Oil Baths

For essential oil baths to achieve specific effects, such as chamomile for relaxation and pain relief, use a few drops of the oil in the bath and soak for up to half an hour. *See* chapter 8 on the properties and indications of aromatic oils, and choose accordingly.

Oatmeal Bath

For an oatmeal bath, ideal for any skin irritations, take 1lb (½ kilo) of uncooked oatmeal and place it in a gauze bag which should be held under a running hot tap, thereby releasing the ingredients which are soothing to the skin. Float the bag in the bath while soaking in it and use it as a sponge to gently pat areas of irritation. The temperature of the bath should be around 96°F (36°C). Stay in the bath for at least 20 minutes. Pat dry afterwards, without rubbing.

Mustard Bath

This is recommended in the early stages of a developing headache.

Materials and method

- One teaspoonful of powdered mustard is added to 2 gallons (9 litres) of hot water in a bowl large enough for both feet to rest in.
- A similar bowl, also containing hot mustard water, rests on the knees, and the hands and forearms are placed in it.
- Put a cool, damp cloth on the forehead.
- After 20 minutes wash the hands and feet thoroughly and rest.

The Moor Bath

When you use a peat-like substance called Moor in a bath you are adding the concentrated natural product of hundreds of thousands of years of compression of the organic materials from decaying mosses, leaves and roots (*see* chapter 8 for more information). The resulting 'soup' contains rich supplies of silica, sulphur, iron, resins and many minerals and harmless acids. Many of these ingredients help to neutralize harmful toxins on and under the skin, and since many of the micro-elements in Moor can be absorbed through the skin, it can also influence your general health. There are particular benefits to skin and rheumatic problems, although medical research has also shown that Moor baths can help blood pressure problems, circulatory difficulties and in restoring balance when there are sugar disturbances.

Materials

• Liquid Moor peat (from pharmacies, drug stores, specialist beauty suppliers or health stores)

Method

The very best way of using Moor is to apply it as a paste to the body surface as a whole, but while this can be done effectively at health spas it is not a practical proposition in the home. By using liquid Moor, home treatment is possible. All you need do is pour the liquid (amounts will be indicated on the container) into a hot bath and soak for between 20 and 30 minutes. You should shower well afterwards and retire to a warm bed. You might expect to perspire more than usual that night and to sleep very well indeed. Have water by your bed to drink in order to make up the liquid lost through sweating, and be prepared to change your sheets next morning.

How often you use this method depends on your needs. If you are rheumatic and have an acidic tendency then a Moor bath every week would be a good idea. If you just want to experience Moor and give your skin a boost, once or twice a month is adequate.

For more on the therapeutic and beauty uses of Moor, mud and clay, *see* chapter 8.

The Epsom Salts Bath and Flotation Tanks

There are few more effective ways of stimulating skin function than by an Epsom salts bath. It dramatically increases elimin-ation through the skin and, as in the case of the Moor bath, is ideal if there is any tendency towards acidity or rheumatic problems, or if there is a need to detox (and this applies to almost everyone nowadays).

CONTRA-INDICATIONS: Anyone with a serious cardiac condition, or diabetes, or who has a skin condition that is 'open' or weeping, should not use this method.

Materials

- Epsom salts (from any good pharmacy or drug store
- Sea salt
- Iodine

Method

Into a comfortably hot bath place 1lb (0.9 kilos) of commercial Epsom salts plus ¼–½lb (0.25 kilos) of sea salt and a dessertspoonful of iodine (use the clear variety to avoid staining the bath). This combination of salts and iodine approximates the constituents of the sea. Lie in the bath (it is quite impossible to wash in this salt mixture) for not less than 10 minutes and not more than 20. Top up with hot water if you stay in beyond 10 minutes to keep the water feeling hot. When you get out do not shower – just towel yourself dry and get into a prewarmed bed.

As with the Moor bath, you should expect to sweat heavily, and to sleep even more heavily. Have water by the bed as you may need to top up the lost liquid. In the morning take a shower and apply a moisturiser to the skin.

It is not recommended that you take an Epsom salts bath more than once a week; once a month is probably the ideal for general detox purposes and stimulation of skin function.

Simulated Flotation Tank

A novel way of achieving deep relaxation involves the so-called flotation tank, in which you are suspended in very buoyant water inside a light-proof tank. The absence of any stimuli has a profoundly calming effect, although some people find the experience claustrophobic.

The method was first developed during the Second World War by Dr John Lilly, who researched the effects of sensory deprivation and found that floating in water without effort, if the eyes are masked from light and the temperature of the water is

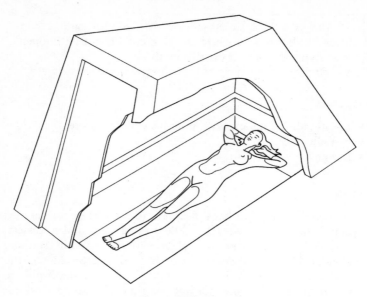

Figure 8 Flotation

neither hot nor cold, produces a profoundly relaxing effect. Anxiety, depression, fatigue and tension, as well as a wide range of painful conditions and even high blood pressure, all responded positively to the method, which evolved into the flotation tank in which you simply float in water saturated with Epsom salts (rather like being in the Dead Sea).

You can approximate the benefits without danger of claustrophobia at home by running an Epsom salts bath with sea salt (as above) at neutral (body heat) temperature, since this equates to the consistency and buoyancy of a flotation tank. Use an eye mask and have some pleasant music in the background, and just lie there for 20 minutes or so, topping up the water with hot when it cools at all.

ADJUNCTIVE HYDROTHERAPY METHODS

Skin Brushing Dry Method

This is best done before you wash, shower or bathe, while your skin is still dry, and it need take only five minutes at most. Once

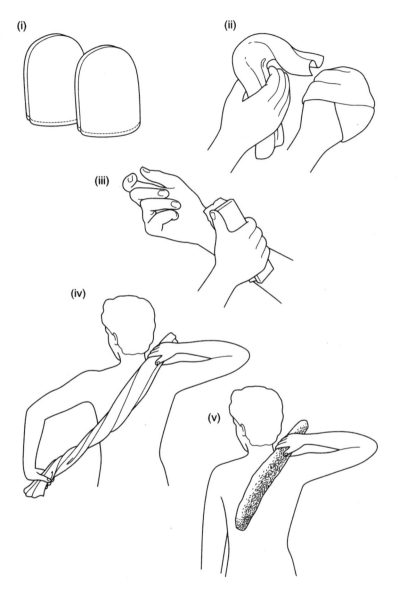

Figure 9 Materials for dry skin brushing can include (i) bath-mitts,
(ii) Flannels, (iii) natural bristle brushes, (iv) rolled towels, and (v) loofahs.

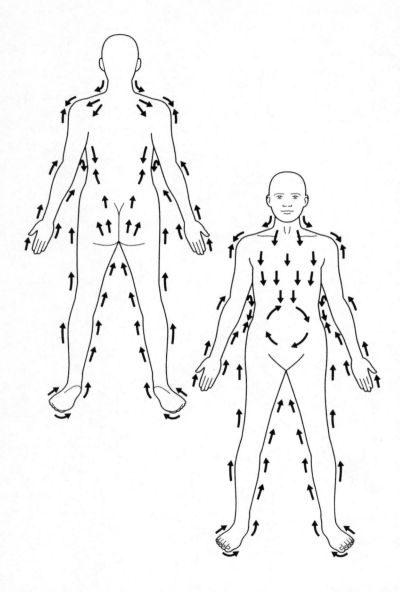

Figure 10 Skin brushing. The body should be brushed in a circular motion to avoid rubbing any one area too much.

you decide to start using skin brushing to improve your skin and health, you should make it a daily routine – and because it makes you feel so good (never mind look good), very soon you will feel as lost without it as you would if you forgot to brush your teeth!

Select from a bath-mitt or a loofah or a natural bristle body-brush. Make sure the room is warm and there are no draughts, because you need to be naked to do this job effectively. It can be done standing, but sitting on a stool allows you to deal with the backs of the legs and other 'difficult' parts more efficiently, without having to perform contortions.

You should start brushing gently. At first expect what is called a 'red reaction', which shows that your circulation is responding to the stimulation you are giving it. The action of brushing needs to be circular, 'creeping', and firm but not irritating. The circular motion helps you avoid rubbing over one area too much – at first once or twice over any part of the skin is adequate. The 'creeping' movement has the same effect; this simply means that you gradually move from where you are circling to the next area, not by lifting the brush, but by altering the direction as you make the circular motion, so sliding gently towards the next part of the skin which is due to receive attention.

Pay particular attention to the skin on the backs of the legs and arms, as well as to your back, abdomen and chest, where you may be more sensitive and tender. Avoid breast tissue, and be very gentle on the inner thighs. If there are bits of your back that you cannot reach, use a dry towel to rub it briskly; it will not be as effective as a brush or loofah, but will be better than no friction at all.

It is emphasized that you should start slowly and gently. After a week or so of skin brushing the skin that was tender will be less so, and you can slowly increase the pressure and vigour of your brushing.

Skin Brushing – Wet Method

To brush using the wet method, choose from the same kinds of brush (bath-mitt or loofah or natural bristle skin-brush). First shower or bathe, and before drying brush the skin as described for dry brushing, but moisten the brush or loofah as well. Shower afterwards, ideally finishing with water that is around body temperature or cooler.

The Salt Glow

The salt glow is basically a skin friction using wet, coarse sea salt or Epsom salts. It is particularly beneficial for people who have difficulty sweating or who have poor circulation to their hands or feet, and is also useful for those prone to rheumatic aches and pains. The salt glow is best done *to* you, and with self-treatment it is necessary to accept that bits of your body are not going to be reached – you can't effectively friction *all* of your back yourself! Unlike skin brushing, which is suggested as a daily routine, the salt glow is a now-and-then thing – perhaps once a week at most if you have difficulty sweating, and once a month or so for general detox purposes.

Materials

- Bowl
- At least ½lb (0.25 kilos) of coarse salt or Epsom salts

Method

Sit on a stool in the bath or shower and add water to the salt in the bowl to moisten it, just enough to make the salt grains stick together. Take a small amount into each hand (approximately a tablespoonful) and starting with one foot work the salt onto the skin as you come up the leg, using up and down and circular motions. Try to friction firmly, even vigorously, on skin that is usually exposed, such as on the legs, so that all the skin gets some rubbing and some salt. Work up each leg and then do each arm. Next work the salt onto the skin around your back without straining yourself (if a partner is there he or she could usefully do this for you). Then apply the salt (rubbing firmly but not irritatingly) to the abdomen and chest and up to the neck, avoiding breast tissue.

After the salt rub you need to shower, ideally using a hand shower and warm water to cleanse the surface of the skin. As the water is playing on each area, use your free hand to rub the salt and water off the skin, giving the area a bit more friction as you do so. Dry with a vigorous towelling down and go to bed – make sure the bed and the room are warm. You should sleep very well. You may perspire heavily the first few times you use the salt glow.

As your skin becomes more efficient, this heavy perspiration will lessen. Have water by the bed in case you get thirsty.

Ice Massage

Ice massage is ideal for acute problems or for regular symptomatic relief of chronic joint problems. Use either ice (messy as it melts) or something metallic that has been in a freezer.

Method

- Empty a soft-drink can of its previous contents, fill it with water and freeze it.
- Seal the hole, and use the can to roll over the painful area to chill it, ensuring that the skin does not frost or become irritated.
- Several minutes of slowly moving iced metal over a joint or other painful area will relieve a good deal of pain.
- If at the same time gentle stretching or painless movement can be introduced, the benefits are enhanced.

Alternatively, try a cold spray such as those used on injuries to reactivate fallen warriors on the sports field. Take care with these sprays as they can blanch and damage the skin, although if used in slow sweeps they are very useful.

Steam Inhalation

Steam penetrates and can be used to reach areas unavailable to any other method, either on its own or as a vehicle for essential oils or herbal essences. Steam inhalation is helpful for:

- painful, tight chest during respiratory infections
- sore throats
- sinus problems

A face sauna or steam-bath opens the pores of the skin and allows for a number of other helpful substances to be absorbed. Follow this with a cold splash and whatever additional skin care you wish to use.

> CONTRA-INDICATIONS: Do not use steam inhalation if there is cardiac asthma or a serious heart condition, or if you are too frail to cope with the heat of steam.

Materials

- Kettle and hot water
- Bowl
- Sheet
- Umbrella, towel or sheet
- Roll of newspaper (optional)
- Essential oils such as eucalyptus or wintergreen, or leaves such as mint (optional)

Method 1

- Bring the kettle to the boil and position it safely near you. Sit close by, covered by a 'tent' made out of the umbrella and draped sheet which also encloses the steaming kettle.
- A few drops of the oil or the leaves of plants can be placed in the kettle and the roll of paper placed over the spout to direct the steam towards your face (this is not essential).
- Breathe the steam slowly and deeply, avoiding any scalding of the skin, which could occur if you are too close to the spout.
- Take great care not to upset the kettle.
- Periodically use a cold damp towel to cool your face and forehead.
- Thirty minutes of steam inhalation, three times daily, helps relieve congestion.

Method 2

- Add boiling water and a few drops of essential oil to a bowl.
- Cover your entire head with a towel and place your face over the steam from the bowl – not too close or you'll irritate your skin – and keep your eyes closed.
- Breathe slowly and deeply for up to 15 minutes or until the steam ceases rising.

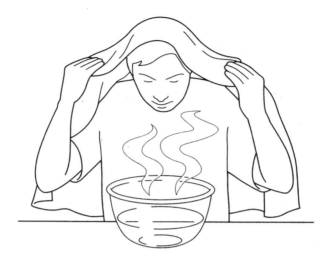

Figure 11 Steam inhalation

Sauna

Unless you are lucky enough to have a sauna at home this needs to be a treat you give yourself at your local health club or sauna bath.

In the wood-lined room of the traditional Scandinavian sauna you are exposed to a dry-heat bath which induces a great deal of perspiration. The effects are profound, and generally include a great deal of tension release and relaxation, along with the enormous elimination produced via the sweating.

The benefits to circulation are well researched and proven, and anyone with a skin problem such as acne can be sure there will be an improvement after the skin has opened in the dry heat. Muscular and joint aches and stiffness are relieved and breathing problems also benefit. Circulation is even further enhanced if the skin is stimulated during the sauna. And you don't have to use birch twigs in the way the Finnish people do – just rub your skin briskly with a loofah or bath-mitt every now and then while sitting in the sauna.

If you are not used to sauna you should stick to a 20-minute introduction followed by a tepid shower (or a cold one – remember the Finns dive into snow after theirs!) and a full body massage. One sauna a month is a wonderful aid to regular detox and skin cleansing – if you have not taken professional advice, and your health is anything other than excellent, saunas should be used cautiously, say (not more than once weekly, in case the process is too exhausting.

Recommended sauna routine

Take a short warm shower followed by 10 to 15 minutes in the sauna, then a 30-second cool or cold plunge (many saunas have plunge baths) or shower. A few minutes rest in the warm room is a good idea at this time. Have another 10 to 15 minutes in the sauna once you are used to the process, followed again by a cool shower or plunge, and a rest. A massage finishes off a super indulgence which will do wonders for you and your skin.

When you are in the sauna you will notice benches, some of which are nearer the ceiling than others, and clearly these are the hottest ones. By adapting to the lower bench first and only moving to the higher ones later you let your body acclimatize to what is a novel experience for most of us.

Don't eat for an hour before or after a sauna, but replenish with liquid whenever you feel the need. Take medical advice before using a sauna if you have any serious medical condition, especially diabetes or heart problems.

Showers

Modern shower heads are remarkably adaptable and capable of producing a wide variety of jets, ranging from a blast to a delicate spray or even an alternating pulsating series of jets. For water therapy in the shower you have a vast range of choices, including:

- Varying the temperature from hot (relaxing) to tepid (very relaxing) to cool or even cold (stimulating and energizing)
- Varying the timing – by keeping the period of heat or cold longer or shorter you can achieve different effects
- Varying the amount of pressure being delivered to the skin by the pressurized shower head
- Using the knowledge of reflex areas to achieve effects in different areas of the body (*see* chapter 3 for details of some reflex pathways)

If you can achieve alternation of temperature quickly, as well as alternation of pressure of water, you have a powerful tool for home hydrotherapy. The benefits include:

- a tonic effect for the circulation (and therefore the skin), which can be general or local
- relaxation or stimulation depending on how you choose to use the shower
- easing of aches and stiffness
- rapid cleansing of the skin and pores

A Hot Shower

Heat relaxes but also enervates or tires you, so do not have a hot shower for a long period (never longer than five minutes) and remember that heat should always be followed by a cool or cold (or at the very least tepid) application of water if you want to help circulation and skin tone. You will clean the skin more effectively with a hot than a cold shower, so use the opportunity to brush vigorously or use a scrub material or wash with pH balanced soap.

If you want to have the hot shower playing onto a stiff or aching area, say your back or a knee, let this be accompanied by placing a cool damp towel on your head while the heat is building in the local area being treated.

A Cold Shower

The effect of cold water is to constrict and contract whatever it is in touch with, so a very brief cold shower, either to finish off after a hot one or on its own, will have an extremely stimulating effect and will actually leave you glowing with inner warmth afterwards, especially if you dry yourself briskly. A minute or two is enough for this effect, and remember that it leads to fewer infections (*see* chapter 1)

The Neutral Shower

Just like the neutral bath or the second stage of the full-sheet pack, a neutral shower (at body heat, so that it feels neither hot nor cold) will have a calming, balancing effect. You can stay in it for as long as you like, even getting a stool into the shower space and sitting there for 10 or 15 minutes if this allows you to become really relaxed.

Alternating Showers

Using alternating hot and cold water allows you to clear the skin, relax the muscles and stimulate the circulation – an amazing series of achievements for just three or four minutes of effort. Start warm and get hotter, taking around one to two minutes to get really hot, then change quickly to a cold shower for 15 seconds, and then go back to hot and then cold, and so on. Or you can stop after one or two alternations if you feel you have done enough for your circulation for one day!

There are no contra-indications. The degree of coldness and hotness you use is up to you and your tolerance. Slowly get yourself to the point where you can not only stand a big contrast (not just going from warm to cool), but actually start to enjoy the thrill of the contrast from hot to cold – and back again.

You can also use the pressure feature of the shower head to play on areas of the body where you feel you need to improve circulation or influence reflex areas.

Enemas and Colonic Irrigations

These methods, which use water and other fluids to wash out either the lower bowel (enema) or the colon as a whole (colonic irrigation), can be extremely useful. They should *not* be used as part of your home health-care programme unless recommended by a health-care professional who understands their use and value, because the delicate flora ('friendly bacteria') of the intestinal tract can be severely depleted and damaged. There is little danger to health if they are used judiciously, but excessive use of these methods is not a good idea.

When they are used their value is enhanced if the water also contains either herbal products to soothe the mucous membrane of the digestive tract (pure aloe vera juice, for example) or friendly bacteria for re-implantation at the end of the procedure.

8

Hydrotherapy Plus – Essential Oils, Moor, Mud and Clay

Combining aspects of aromatherapy with hydrotherapy makes perfect sense as the qualities of the herbal extracts used along with the benefits of appropriate hydrotherapy offer a double benefit.

ESSENTIAL OILS

The use of essential oils is derived from the experience of many aromatherapists and herbal practitioners, and they are safe if used as indicated. The oils described here include the most useful and popular ones for self-massage or for adding to baths, but there are dozens more to try. They can be used to alleviate very real health problems or just to help you feel better or, in a few cases, to look better – choose whatever is applicable to you. When added to a bath the oils are used neat in the running water which disperses them.

Essential oils are widely available from pharmacies, drug stores and health-food stores. Store them individually or in combinations, tightly capped in clean glass containers (dark if possible) away from light.

Basil   Antiseptic, antidepressant and a tonic for the digestion. On its own it can be used to treat weakness, physical and mental fatigue, headaches, nausea, tension, faintness and depression.

Bay   Antiseptic, tonic and decongestant. On its own it can be used to treat colds.

Chamomile Soothing, sleep enhancer, digestive and general tonic, pain reliever and antibacterial. It can be used on its own to treat sleep and digestive disturbances, skin conditions, neuralgia, and inflammation. It soothes tired and irritated eyes when used as a compress or eyewash.

Clove Antiseptic, a stimulant for mind and body, and a reliever of spasm and pain. Used alone it can be helpful for infections, general tension and weakness. It makes a good mouthwash (two drops in a tumbler of water) and is magical as a reliever of toothache when applied neat (in very small amounts on the tip of a cotton-wool stick) to the offending tooth or gum.

Cypress Astringent, antispasmodic, tonic and useful as a deodorant. It can be used alone to treat rheumatic and muscular conditions, coughs, flu and nervous tension.

Eucalyptus Antiseptic, stimulant, insect repellent. It can be used alone to treat flu, sinus infections, laryngitis, breathing problems and coughs, rheumatism and open wounds.

Geranium Tonic and stimulant of adrenalin, astringent, insect repellent and pain reliever. It can be used alone to combat neuralgia, slow healing of wounds and burns, and for poor circulation. It acts as a skin tonic.

Juniper Nerve tonic, diuretic, and digestive aid. It is used alone to treat indigestion, nervous conditions, fluid retention, rheumatism and some skin conditions (it is antifungal).

Lavender Antispasmodic, antiseptic, general restorative, insect repellent. It can be used alone to treat nervous problems and skin lesions such as burns, wounds and acne. It makes a useful douche. Use a few drops neat on minor burns (although always call a doctor if burns are serious).

Lemon Tonic, antiseptic, diuretic, insect repellent. It can be used alone to treat rheumatic problems, digestive upsets, gout, fluid retention and poor skin tone.

Marjoram Stimulant and tonic. Combine marjoram with

ylang-ylang – six drops of each in 4fl oz (114ml) of carrier oil – for massage in cases of depression.

Neroli Antidepressant, antiseptic, digestive aid, sedative, aphrodisiac. Used alone it can treat depression, insomnia and nervous tension, digestive upsets and lack of sexual interest. It is a skin-enhancing agent.

Peppermint Stimulant for the nervous system, digestive aid, antispasmodic, pain reliever, insect repellent. Use it alone to treat fatigue, indigestion, migraine and breathing problems, including asthma.

Pine Antiseptic, diuretic and tonic (stimulates adrenalin production). It is used alone to treat infections, fluid retention, rheumatic conditions, coughs, colds and fatigue, and together with eucalyptus for bronchitis, coughs and sinus problems.

Rose Antibacterial, antidepressant, aphrodisiac, astringent, sedative, tonic for the heart and liver. It has specific influences on the female reproductive organs, especially the uterus. Alone it is used to treat depression, poor sex drive, headache, nausea and insomnia, as well as being useful for douching and as a skin tonic.

Rosemary Stimulant of hormones from the adrenal glands, antiseptic and decongestant. Applications on its own include treatment of colds and infections, rheumatic and gout-related conditions, burns and sores on the skin, fatigue and excess fat in the tissues.

Sage Tonic, antiseptic, diuretic, with influences on the female reproductive system and blood pressure. Alone it is used to treat nervousness, fatigue, chest complaints, menopausal problems and low blood pressure, and it is useful as a douche.

Sandalwood Antiseptic, aphrodisiac and tonic. It is used alone to treat bronchitis, urinary infections, impotence and fatigue.

Tea Tree Antiseptic, antifungal.

Thyme General stimulant, antiseptic, antispasmodic and neutralizer of snake venom. It is used alone to treat tiredness, digestive

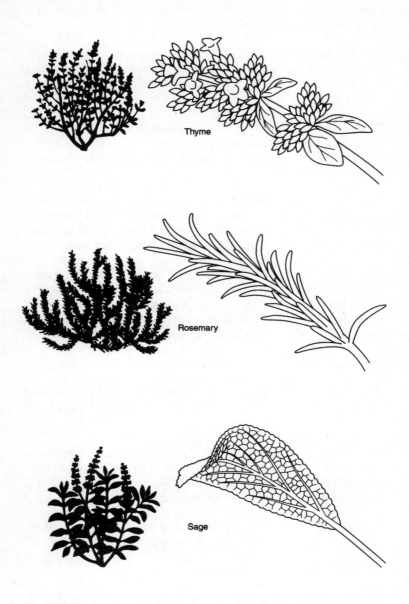

Figure 12 Herbs for essential oils

problems, infections, rheumatic conditions, inflammation of the skin, intestinal parasites and snakebite.

Vetiver   This is a calming agent and is used to treat anxiety and nervous conditions. Combine it with lavender for anxiety and tension.

Ylang-Ylang   Sedative, antiseptic, aphrodisiac. Its use alone is for treatment of high blood pressure, intestinal infections and impotence. Use it with marjoram for depression.

Summary of Conditions and Appropriate Essential Oils (for external use only)

Acne – cypress, lemon, lavender, tea tree
Anxiety – basil, lavender, neroli, vetiver
Arthritis – chamomile, eucalyptus, rosemary, sandalwood
Bites and stings – basil, lavender, marjoram, thyme
Bladder problems – eucalyptus, juniper, sandalwood, thyme
Bronchial problems – eucalyptus, pine, sandalwood
Burns (minor) – lavender
Cellulite – juniper, marjoram, rosemary, thyme
Chronic fatigue – geranium, juniper, lavender, rosemary
Colds – eucalyptus, pine, sandalwood
Depression – basil, marjoram, neroli, ylang-ylang
Dry skin – lavender, rose, sandalwood
Fever – eucalyptus, lavender, peppermint
Fungal infections – tea tree, lavender
Gout – juniper, rosemary
Haemorrhoids – chamomile, cypress, lavender, juniper
Hair loss – bay, lavender
Headache – chamomile, lavender, peppermint, rosemary
Indigestion – basil, chamomile, peppermint
Insect repellent – clove, eucalyptus, geranium, lemon
Menopausal problems – chamomile, cypress, lavender, sage
Menstrual cramping – chamomile, cypress, marjoram, sage
Migraine headaches – cypress, lavender, rosemary, sage
Rheumatism – chamomile, eucalyptus, rosemary, sandalwood
Sinus problems – cypress, eucalyptus, pine
Sunburn – chamomile, lavender
Varicose veins – cypress, geranium

THE THERAPEUTIC AND BEAUTY USES OF MOOR, MUD AND CLAY

'Mud, mud, glorious mud, nothing quite like it for cooling the blood' ... well, maybe for a hippo, but what about you? The truth is that mud is a most amazing conglomeration of ingredients and it can be remarkably health enhancing when used correctly. We will look briefly at just three of the most researched and useful examples of mud, clay and peat, from Austria, Israel and France – there are many others.

Austrian Moor Products

Analysis of the extraordinary 'Moor' mud-like substance from Austria ('Neydharting Moor') shows that it contains an enormous variety of organic and inorganic minerals, oils, proteins, wax, resins, saturated and unsaturated fats, useful acids, natural antibiotics and vitamins.

The Austrians say categorically that this is *not* peat – peat, they explain, is the product of decaying trees which have been submerged in water for thousands of years. In the absence of air, the trees rot down and the end result is largely cellulose derived from wood fibre. Moor, on the other hand, is the result of chemical, biological and biochemical changes in medicinal herbs and other plants including their roots, leaves, stalks, blooms, fruits, seeds and tubers. Over 1,000 different plants have been identified in the Austrian Moor products, 300 of which have medicinal value, and 200 of which have been extinct for over 500 years. These medicinal plants and their trace elements, vitamins, plant hormones, plant antibiotics (to protect the plant against infection) and unique plant oils and wax, are preserved forever in the Moor.

It is estimated that Neydharting Moor material is around 20,000 years old and its therapeutic use dates back to before Roman times when the Celts first used it in 800 BC. The 16th-century physician Paracelsus wrote of its value, and the 'Moor Cure' was taken by King Louis XV and his Court, as well as by Napoleon and Josephine.

Modern research has now shown it to have enormous therapeutic value. It is an astringent, it is absorbent of toxic body wastes, acid-balancing (ion-exchanging) and anti-inflammatory.

The various ingredients of Moor penetrate the skin, improving its tone and circulation, as well as entering the body itself. Moor products are available from many health stores, drug stores and pharmacies.

Neydharting Moor life soap

This maintains skin acidity at its optimum level and is ideal for normal cosmetic use and for sensitive or damaged skin.

Neydharting Moor life-cleansing and toning lotion

This is claimed to be ideal for either oily or dry and sensitive skin. It actively discourages acne and enhances skin tone, helping to restore and maintain skin acidity (pH) levels. There is also a Moor face cream and body cream.

Neydharting Moor life mask

This is made up of the essence of 20,000-year-old flowers, plants, grasses and herbs. Its essential oils and lipids penetrate easily into the skin and have a cleansing and rejuvenating effect. It is unperfumed and perhaps not too glamorous when applied as a mask, but the results are what counts. Wash your face using Moor soap. Place a little of the mask material into an egg cup and add a teaspoon of water. Mix until the material 'hangs' on to the skin of your fingers, not slipping off too easily. Apply the paste to the face with fingers or a brush and leave it on for three minutes if you have dry skin, or up to eight minutes if you have 'problem' skin. Wash the face mask off with warm water and apply the Moor cleansing and toning cream, followed if you wish by the Moor face cream. This process is recommended once a week for normal skin, and daily for up to three weeks and twice a week thereafter for problem skins.

Moor life bath

This is taken at body temperature (a neutral bath) for about 20 minutes. The liquid ingredients are a mix of water and the Moor extract. No washing takes place in these baths – just lie and relax, and when leaving the bath pat yourself dry. The material will continue to be active for hours after the bath. The indications for using a Moor bath include rheumatism, arthritis, detox, hormonal and menstrual difficulties and skin problems including eczema, psoriasis and acne. Full instructions as to quantity are given on every bottle, but the basic amount of Moor used is roughly ½ pint (around a fifth of a litre) in each bath.

Drinking the Moor material

Odd as it may seem, the herbal constituents of the product make Moor suitable for oral use.

Neydharting Moor life herbal drink

This is extracted from the Moor material and is useful for a variety of disorders including rheumatic and arthritic problems, and digestive and intestinal problems including gallstones. It is ideal for use in any detox programme and for anyone with a sensitive digestion and tendency to liverish symptoms. It is suggested that it be taken three times daily for between four and six weeks to be most effective

Dead Sea Products

Romantic Biblical and historical figures such as the Queen of Sheba, Cleopatra, King Solomon and King David are all said to have had curative bathing palaces on the Dead Sea in ancient times. The Dead Sea (really a vast inland lake) and its adjacent hot springs differ from all other known bodies of water in that the exceptionally high concentrations of mineral salts (nearly 28 per cent – four times more than sea water) make the water so dense that you cannot sink in it; it supports your weight fully. Chemical analysis of water and mud from this lowest place on the planet (it is nearly 1,300ft (400 m) below sea level) reveals an enormous content of minerals including iodine, bromine, chloride, carbonic acid, sulphates, sodium, potassium, calcium, magnesium, lithium, strontium, hydrogen sulphide and radium.

Apart from having remarkable (and well-researched) healing effects on skin conditions such as psoriasis, the Dead Sea products that are now available have a wide range of applications for health and beauty enhancement. Any home health spa should have them in stock.

The Dead Sea range of products also includes scalp and general body applications for different types of skin and for many different health problems. These include baths, mud packs for the face, exfoliant creams, lotions and moisturizers for body and face, day and night creams and ointments. They are available from many health stores, drug stores and pharmacies.

Dead Sea mineral salts bath

The producers of Dead Sea products recommend that anyone with rheumatic or arthritic or general aches, pains and stiffness take a series of lukewarm baths (around 98.6°F (37°C) or up to 104°F (40°C) if you have rheumatic pain) into which a pack of the salt is dissolved; you can use up to two packs for a more powerful salt bath. You are recommended to soak for between half an hour and an hour in the water before towelling dry and applying a mineral-rich Dead Sea moisturizing agent.

The main indications are for alleviation of aches and pains, whether muscular or joint, as well as for skin conditions such as eczema and psoriasis. If there are health problems of this sort three or four treatments weekly for a month are recommended.

These Dead Sea salt baths are completely safe and no side effects should be anticipated.

Mud mask

The black mud from the Dead Sea contains over 20 minerals and trace elements, many of which are absorbed through the skin on application as a facial mask. The effect is to exfoliate (remove dead skin), to draw impurities through the skin and to increase local circulation.

French Clay

Clay is a most remarkable natural substance, with the power to absorb and retain toxic materials. It is used in industry on an enormous scale. This ability to draw into itself, and to hold fast to, toxic matter means that when clay is used for health or beauty purposes, internally or externally, it has to be drawn from very pure unpolluted sites. This is why French clay is usually mined from a depth of just under 200ft (60m) or more along the banks of pristine rivers, usually in wooded areas. The sand-free clay is then sun-dried before packing.

The chemical composition of pure clay includes large quantities of silica, iron, calcium, magnesium, zinc and enzymes. The French use the clay internally for general and specific health enhancement, by stirring a teaspoon (child's dose) or two (adult dose) of the powdered material into a glass of water and drinking it, a method that has profound detox potential as the clay passes through the digestive tract. It is not absorbed, although any minerals within it may be.

Among conditions that have been shown to benefit from clay are rheumatism, allergy, asthma, stomach discomfort, food poisoning, chronic inflammation of the digestive tract, headaches, and hyperactivity in children if this is related to food intolerance.

Using clay externally

For purification of the skin a face mask of green clay (for general use) or yellow clay (if there are skin problems as it contains sulphur) is ideal. Clay absorbs impurities, cleansing the skin and promoting circulation.

The mask can be prepared from the powdered clay by mixing it with water before application, or directly from a tube which is pre-mixed. Pre-mixed clay is also ideal as first aid for treating bites and stings, as well as for local application to sprains and bruises.

Green clay, the most common one, comes in the form of chunks, or bars which need to be broken up, and in this form it has to be soaked in water for about two hours before it achieves the pliable consistency needed for use. Green clay is also marketed in very fine powdered form ready for use once mixed with water (preferably pure spring water).

Clay should be applied to painful areas such as joints or muscles in a layer just under 1 inch thick and immediately covered with a muslin or cotton cloth. This poultice should be left in place for not less than an hour and ideally overnight. When removed the 'used' clay should be disposed of and never reused as it will contain appreciable levels of toxins that have been drawn through the skin.

Variations on green clay include:

- White superfine clay for internal use as described, especially for those with a sensitive digestion, and for external use as a powder for irritated skin
- Yellow extra-fine clay for internal use for people with poor metabolism, and for external use as a paste for skin impurities
- Red superfine clay for use internally for those who are fatigued

French products are available from specialized health stores, pharmacies, drug stores and beauty salons.

9

Detox

Some of the hydrotherapy measures detailed in this book, including:

Constitutional hydrotherapy
Epsom salts bath
Full-sheet pack
Various essential oil baths
Heating compress (on trunk to cover liver area)

– have the potential to encourage detoxification.

WHY SHOULD WE NEED TO 'DETOX'?

The normal functions of life produce toxins all the time. The waste products of metabolism (the multiple processes going on constantly within us) form as our bodies create energy, digest food, transport blood or work muscles. When we are healthy these toxins are usually eliminated or neutralized by processes taking place in organs such as the liver, kidneys, bowels, lungs and, most importantly, the skin.

The toxins are created more rapidly and cleared more slowly when we are stressed. For example, tense muscles create and retain acid wastes. These acid wastes can be flushed away by exercise and fresh, oxygenated blood, and can also be excreted through the skin as sweat; or they can be retained in the tissues due to sluggish circulation and poor oxygenation as a result of inadequate exercise and breathing. If toxins are not efficiently eliminated they become irritants and interfere with normal function. Reducing tension and performing regular exercise and deep breathing, as well as introducing methods – such as hydrotherapy – for increasing elimination through the skin will reduce part of the toxic burden.

All our organs of detoxification need to be well nourished in order to work efficiently. This means our organs and tissues need to be well supplied with fresh, oxygenated blood carrying adequate nutrient supplies, and served by a nervous system that is working correctly. As we get older, and as we are exposed to a greater degree of toxicity and stress from many sources, so our ability to self-cleanse – to detox – becomes less efficient, as do our various supporting functions such as circulation and elimination. Because of atmospheric, water and food pollution we all now carry within ourselves a cocktail of chemicals derived from solvents, pesticides, food additives, petrochemical by-products and heavy metals. If we do not eliminate these toxins efficiently we retain this undesirable debris stored in our tissues, mainly in the fat below our skin. This is added to daily by exposure to new toxic materials in our food, water and the air we breathe, not to forget any extra toxicity we create or acquire through infection or from certain forms of medication.

No one has a clear idea of just what damage all this is doing to us, especially if you consider the combination of these toxic burdens interacting with the individual biochemical differences we are born with. We also all have huge differences in our levels of nutritional, structural and emotional excellence or deficiency. Some of us handle the toxic load better than others, but in the end all of us are negatively affected by toxicity – sometimes with profound consequences to the levels of health we enjoy, or the sort and intensity of the illnesses we suffer.

Good News

The need to tackle these toxic burdens before they actually show up as ill health has never been greater – the good news is that there is an enormous amount we can do to help ourselves. Not only can we try to ensure a balanced diet, but we can make sure we get enough of the right sort of exercise. We can also take care of that vital area which controls everything else – our emotional and stress coping functions – and we can work at regularly cleansing our system, with hydrotherapy as a key part of this process.

Many scientists believe that in the future health care will have at its very core an absolute requirement for safe and effective detox procedures. These procedures can and hopefully will be started before our immune system and vital organs have started to decline in efficiency. A healthy immune system, efficient organs of elimination and detoxification and a sound circulatory and nervous system can handle a great deal of toxicity. Supporting these functions, organs and systems – either because we want to keep them well and efficient, or because they may have shown signs that they are not operating optimally – is one of the best arguments for regularly using water therapy along with other self-help methods such as improved diet and exercise patterns.

In order to get a picture of your current needs in detox terms it is worth assessing your current state of 'toxicity' and health by answering the questions on the following pages.

DO YOU NEED TO DETOX?

There are several questions in this section to help you identify where to place the emphasis in your health enhancement campaign. Obviously if we were all to eat a balanced diet and relax and exercise sufficiently, while carefully avoiding exposure to toxins, we would all be healthier – but most of us don't and aren't.

And to confuse the whole scene it is now well established that what makes a perfectly balanced diet for you may not suit me; that I might need a great deal more (or less) exercise to stay fit than you do; and that because of where and how we were born and raised, and our respective parents' health status, and the many different things to which we have been exposed since childhood, you and I might carry quite different toxic 'burdens' in our systems and be able to cope (or not cope) with stress in quite different ways. It is important to identify your particular need for detoxification, whether you may be nutritionally deficient, or over stressed or under exercised.

The questionnaires on the following pages give guidelines only; they are not meant to take the place of responsible medical assessment or care. They provide evidence of tendencies and possibilities, not certainties. If they raise doubts in your mind please discuss these with a professional health adviser. The real aim of the questions is to guide you in making choices between the many options that are open to you.

Are You Nutritionally Deficient?

The following signs can indicate nutrient deficiency, which can mean that the particular nutrient is not forming a sufficient part of your diet, or that you are not absorbing and/or utilizing the nutrients you are eating. Either way, nutrient deficiency can impact considerably onto your general health and your body's ability to handle toxins.

Do you have	**Possible deficiency**
A poor sense of smell and/or taste?	Zinc
Hair which is falling out or breaks easily?	Protein
A very red or sensitive tongue?	Vitamin B complex
Whites of eyes which are slightly blue?	Iron and/or Vit C
Gums which bleed on cleaning?	Zinc and/or Vit C.
Cramps at night?	Calcium/Magnesium
Cuts which heal only slowly?	Zinc and/or Vit C
Rough skin on elbows or knees?	Vitamin A
Trouble seeing at twilight?	Vitamin A
Red, greasy and scaly skin on the face or nose?	Vitamin B2
Seborrhoeic dermatitis on the face or nose?	Vitamin B6
Cracking at the corners of the mouth?	Vitamins B2, B6 or folic acid

A balanced diet (see below) will help to sort out these sorts of imbalance naturally. Supplementation of vitamins should be undertaken after taking responsible advice from a health-care professional.

Should You Detox?

1 Do you drink more than one and a half glasses of wine, or one pint of beer, or any spirits daily? (YES scores 3 points)

2　Do you drink more than a single cup each of coffee or tea daily? (YES scores 3 points)

3　Do you eat or drink chocolate or drink cola more than once a week? (YES scores 3 points)

4　Do you drink tap water or use it in cooking or when making drinks? (YES scores 3 points)

5　Do you eat smoked, preserved or barbecued foods more than once a week? (YES scores 3 points)

6　Do you eat mainly 'normal' (not organically grown) vegetables and fruit? (YES scores 3 points)

7　If you do eat 'normal' fruits do you eat the skin (apples, pears, and so on)? (YES scores 3 points)

8　If you eat 'normal' vegetables do you wash them well and scrub and peel root vegetables to eliminate chemical residues? (NO scores 3 points)

9　Do you eat mainly 'normal' (not free range) meat, poultry and eggs? (YES scores 3 points)

10　Do you eat foods more than once a week which contain colouring, preservatives or other additives? (YES scores 3 points)

11　Have you taken prescription medication for depression, anxiety or sleep disturbance for more than a month in the past year?

12　Have you had an amalgam filling in your teeth within the last year, or do you have more than two amalgams in your mouth?

13　Do you smoke, live with a smoker, or take 'recreational drugs'?

14　Do you live or work near heavy industrial factories, a main traffic thoroughfare, or in a double-glazed office environment, or are you regularly exposed to or in contact with toxic fumes or chemicals of any sort?

If you score over 12, or answer YES to questions 11, 12, 13 or 14, you are in need of some of the gentle detox methods described in this book. We can all benefit from periodic detox, whatever our present health status.

Exercise and Lifestyle

How we structure our daily routine has a powerful influence on our health, and this includes exercise (or lack of it) and a host of less obvious factors on which the questions below will help you focus.

1 Do you work (in the home or out of it) for more than 40 hours a week?

2 Do you regularly work for more than 10 hours on any given day?

3 Do you spend less than half an hour over your main meals?

4 Do you eat quickly, not chewing adequately?

5 Do you get less than 7 hours sleep in 24?

6 Do you spend some time, regularly, listening to relaxing music?

7 Do you regularly practise some form of relaxation?

8 Do you get at least half an hour's active exercise three times a week?

9 Do you enjoy a creative hobby (gardening, painting, music, and so on) and spend time on this regularly?

10 Do you perform some sort of non-competitive activity such as yoga, tai chi, cycling or swimming?

11 Do you have regular bodywork treatment for relaxation (osteopathy, massage, aromatherapy, reflexology)?

12 Do you get outside in the fresh air in daylight for at least half an hour each day?

The answers to questions 1 to 5 should be NO, and if they are currently YES you should try to modify the situation to turn them into NO answers over a period of time.

The answers to questions 6 to 12 should all be YES, and if they are currently NO you should try to modify them slowly towards YES.

The answers to all these questions will also give you pointers to your body's ability to detox naturally.

AN UNBALANCED DIET – THE ENEMY OF HEALTH AND BEAUTY

Diet, Illness and Ageing

One important and little understood aspect of how diet influences not just health but appearance as well involves some minute 'rogue' molecules called free radicals, which set up a chemical process known as oxidation. This is one of the major causes of ageing and especially of one of its least attractive aspects – wrinkles.

When hair is bleached the change in colour is caused by oxidation. The same process takes place when metal rusts or tarnishes, when rubber perishes, when fats or oils become rancid or when a potato or apple turns brown when cut in half. It also happens inside you and me, all the time, because oxidation is one of the ways in which your immune system protects you from harmful bacteria. Your defence cells actually manufacture tiny amounts of hydrogen peroxide to kill them. But while oxidation can be a useful natural process, it can also be damaging. Oxidation is thought to be one of the main ways in which arthritis, hardening of the arteries and cancer begin, as well as being a major part of the ageing process.

What causes oxidation?

Every atom (you and everything else on this planet are made up of atoms linked together into molecules) has in orbit around it minute negatively and positively charged electrons and protons. They are usually balanced in pairs, making them stable. For example, when one oxygen atom joins with two hydrogen atoms we get a water molecule, H_2O, a stable substance with no 'free' electrons.

If, however, we have two hydrogen atoms and two oxygen atoms joined together we get H_2O_2 (hydrogen peroxide, or bleach), which has free electrons and is therefore a free radical. A free radical is dangerous because its free electron causes it to behave like a violent football hooligan, grabbing electrons from any passing substance with which it comes into contact. If a stable molecule has an electron ripped away by a free radical it becomes unstable itself, and it will then try to hijack an electron from somewhere else.

Free radicals and our bodies

When our defence systems manufacture free radicals to kill invading germs, they do it in such small amounts that damage seldom results in our own tissues, so this is not the source of dangerous levels of free radicals. One source may actually be your own tissues! Much of the material that makes up your body cells consists of lipid or fatty substances and these, like all fats, are likely under the wrong conditions to become oxidized.

Another source of free radicals is heavy metals, such as lead and cadmium, which are found in polluted air and water and which we all have inside our tissues as part of our toxic burden. Other toxic substances that cause free radical activity include tobacco smoke (which has high levels of cadmium and other free radical containing elements) and by-products of the petro-chemical industry found in the air we breathe or in our water supply. When 'wrong' conditions occur (too much fatty tissue and/or heavy metal toxicity), free radicals are most active and the chain reaction of oxidation begins.

Stopping the damage

Oxidation starts and goes on until substances called antioxidants come along to quench the process, just like putting out a fire (which is itself an example of free radical activity on a grand scale). Violent free radical behaviour is therefore controllable by a 'fire brigade' made up of antioxidant substances. For example, when, in a smoke-filled room, your eyes start to sting, this is because of free radical activity irritating the surface of your eyes. The tears that follow contain glutathione peroxidase, a strong antioxidant enzyme, which quenches and stops this process.

It is always better to prevent something rather than trying to stop it once it has started. So a squeeze of lemon (antioxidant) on a cut apple stops it turning brown (oxidizing), thanks to vitamin C. Antioxidants are what we use to rust-proof metal or stop it from tarnishing. They also preserve oils and fats in food from going rancid, and they can preserve us from the worst effects of the ageing process.

Protection is therefore available from eating antioxidant-rich foods. Antioxidants are found most plentifully in fresh fruit and vegetables, which is one reason for the medical emphasis on high levels of them in our diets. Antioxidants include vitamins A, C and E, and a trio of anti-ageing, protective enzymes – superoxide dismutase, catalase and glutathione peroxidase – found in young sprouting plants, many fresh fruits (especially papaya, mango, pineapple, kiwi fruit and berries) and salad vegetables.

We gain a lot of these enzymes by eating such foods, or by supplementing ourselves with freeze-dried juice from sprouting plants such as wheat, which is particularly rich in them. General 'insurance' supplementation of antioxidants is easy thanks to products that combine the best of them, including vitamins A, C, E and selenium. Powerful plant-based antioxidant enzymes, as mentioned above, are also available for those who wish to boost protection even more.

The best approach, of course, is to avoid contact with free radicals if possible – stick to fresh air, clean pure water, no smoking – and to boost natural antioxidant intake through fresh food, preferably raw or lightly cooked. If you are really aiming for high-level well-being, energy galore and eyes and skin that express the inner health you have created, then a diet that provides all your nutrients in an easily digested form is your best approach. In addition, the detox diet outlined below gives you a wonderful opportunity to minimize the damage caused by oxidation. You should be able to build this into your normal routine without difficulty.

A Gentle Detox Programme

Before deciding to detox get advice from a health professional to help you select the degree of intensity with which you should apply the various methods available. If you are robust and vital a more vigorous programme will be appropriate than if you are unwell or your health is fragile. Are you well enough to undertake rapid and active detox, or is it better to string the process out in order to do the job slowly? Whichever is better for you, the ingredients of the detox programme are the same – it's only the speed and strength of what is done that needs to be modified according to individual needs.

The following detox programme is safe for almost everyone, but if you are a recovering drug user or alcoholic, or have an eating disorder or are a diabetic, then do not apply these methods without asking professional advice first.

Priority number one in detoxification is dietary. Choose

between the following detox diets over almost every weekend for a few months, and thereafter once a month at least.

Short water-only fast

This lasts for 24 to 36 hours, either starting Friday evening and ending Saturday evening, or just all day Saturday so that work schedules are not interfered with. Make sure that you consume not less than 4 pints (2 litres) and not more than 8 pints (4 litres) of water during the day. On the Sunday have a raw food day, with fruit and salad only, well chewed, plus as much water as you like.

Full weekend monodiet

Start on Friday night and go through to Sunday evening on a single food. You can have up to 3lbs (1.4 kilos) daily of a single fruit such as grapes, apples, pears (the best choice if an allergy history exists) or papaya (ideal if digestive problems exist); or brown rice, buckwheat or millet; or potatoes (skin and all), boiled and eaten whenever desired. You can eat up to 1lb (0.45 kilos) dry weight of any of the grains (made palatable by the addition of a little lemon juice and olive oil) or 3lb (1.4 kilos) of potatoes daily.

Whichever type of weekend detox you choose make sure you rest and keep warm and have no engagements – this is a time to allow all available energy to focus on the repairing and cleansing processes of detox.

Midweek detox diet

In between these weekend detox intensives, a milder midweek programme will boost your health still more.

Breakfast   Choose between the following:

- fresh fruit (raw or lightly cooked, with no sweetening) and live yogurt
- home-made muesli (seeds and nuts and grains) and live yogurt
- cooked grains (such as buckwheat, millet, linseed, barley and rice) and yogurt

Drink   Herbal tea (linden blossom, chamomile, mint, sage, lemon verbena) or a lemon and hot water drink.

Lunch and supper One of these should be a raw salad with jacket potato or brown rice and either bean curd (tofu) or low-fat cheese or nuts and seeds. Or, if raw food is a problem, a stir-fried vegetable and tofu meal, or steamed vegetables eaten with potato or rice together with low-fat cheese or nuts and seeds.

The other main meal should be a choice between fish, chicken, game or vegetarian savoury (a pulse and grain combination) and vegetables lightly steamed, baked or stir-fried.

Desserts Lightly stewed fruit (add apple or lemon juice, not sugar) or live natural yogurt.

Season food with garlic and herbs, avoiding salt as much as possible. Eat slowly, chew well, don't drink with meals and consume at least 2 pints (1 litre) of liquid daily between meals. Also take one high-potency multimineral/multivitamin capsule daily and three garlic capsules, along with an acidophilus supplement for bowel detox support.

ADDITIONAL DETOX SUPPORT

The treatments described throughout this book will aid your detox programme. They include:

- Epsom salt baths or wet-sheet packs – once weekly
- Constitutional hydrotherapy – alternate days
- Skin brushing to assist skin elimination function – daily
- Stretching and relaxation exercises – daily
- If appropriate, brisk aerobic exercise (walking, jogging, skipping, rebounding, dancing, workout) – every day except during the fasting period
- Massage and lymphatic drainage massage as often as available – twice weekly if possible
- Use of appropriate essential aromatherapy oils in baths or as part of massage
- Breathing, relaxation and meditation methods – every day at least once for 10–15 minutes, and preferably twice.

What to Expect

In the early days (the first few weekends) you could develop a headache and furred tongue – don't worry. It will slowly get less obvious as detox progresses. Take nothing to stop the headache, just rest as much as you can.

As the weeks pass your skin and eyes should become clearer (although your skin may get a bit spotty for a while), your brain sharper, your digestion more efficient, your energy levels should rise and you should regain a feeling of youthful clarity.

When your tongue no longer becomes furred with the weekend detox and headaches no longer appear, you can begin to spread these intensive detox weekends apart – three a month, then two a month, and then maintenance of once a month. The in-between pattern can also be relaxed a bit, with the inclusion of a few 'naughty but nice' tasty toxins from time to time. By this time your internal detox system should be able to cope with such indiscretions – enjoy!

10

Exercise and Stress Relief

Hydrotherapy works wonders, but it is important to include it into a comprehensive approach to health enhancement. This means taking into account your lifestyle habits, especially exercise and stress levels.

EXERCISE – IN AND OUT OF WATER

There are two key forms of exercise that are important if you are to get the most out of home hydrotherapy programmes. One involves active movement, using the aerobic principle, and the other involves slow, stretching movements, such as those involved in yoga and tai chi. One without the other will result in imbalance: to have healthy, 'fit' muscles which are also pliable you need to use both.

Your Aerobic Index

In order to achieve aerobic conditions effectively, and so tone circulation and heart function, you have to exercise neither too strenuously nor too gently. There is a mathematical formula that can tell you how much you need to do to really get the most benefit. Working out your 'aerobic index' is therefore desirable, but it is not essential. If you want to be unstructured in your exercising, without any feeling of having to check your pulse periodically to see whether you are doing 'enough' or 'too much', then forget the formula and just do as much as you want to – it might be all you need. If, however, you want to do what the professionals do, calculating your 'aerobic index' is certainly the best choice.

- The first step is to have a watch with a second hand, plus a pencil and paper, by your bed to check your resting pulse on waking in the morning. Before getting up, take your pulse for a full minute and record it. Do the same three mornings running, then add the three numbers together and divide by three to get an average resting pulse rate.
- Let's say your resting pulse rate is 70. Add this number to your age. Let's say this is 40.
- 70 + 40 = 110
- Take that number away from 220:
- 220 – 110 = 110
- You are now required to do some serious arithmetic. You need to know what 60 per cent and 80 per cent of the latest figure (110) are:
- 110 ÷ 10 = 11, × 6 = 66
- 110 ÷ 10 = 11, × 8 = 88
- Now you need to *add back* your morning pulse average:
- 66 + 70 = 136
- 88 + 70 = 158

These are the important safety numbers for aerobics for anyone whose age is 40 and whose morning resting pulse rate is 70. Remember this is an example only – to find the index you need to apply you must use *your own* resting pulse rate and *your own* age.

When you are exercising you need to check your pulse rate periodically – say every five minutes – to make sure that it stays *above* the lower figure (136 in this example) for 20 minutes not less than three times a week.

It is necessary to keep this going for at least 20 minutes three times a week in order to achieve an aerobic effect which ensures greater fitness and cardiovascular efficiency. And of course you must make sure that your active pulse rate *stays below* 158 (in this same example), so that you avoid any risk to heart function.

When you check your pulse while exercising do so for only 10 seconds and multiply by 6 (to get the rate for a full minute); if you stop to take your pulse for too long the aerobic effect can be lost.

It isn't surprising that many people can't be bothered to do all this, although once you have done the arithmetic the rest is simple. If you opt simply to get regular exercise without knowing what your pulse is doing, don't feel guilty – we are not all made the same way! But if you *do* choose to follow these guidelines, remember that as you get fitter month by month you need to recheck your morning pulse rate – it might have gone down, meaning that you need to do less to achieve the aerobic effect. And, of course, the sums need to be done again each year as you get older.

What sort of exercise you opt for is up to you. Whether you skip or use a rebounder (mini-trampoline) or dance to jazz music, or do ballet, or run or jog or walk or swim or play a competitive sport, it's all the same to your cardiovascular system. Our particular focus is water therapy, and so in this instance these figures need to be viewed in relation to exercise in water.

Important things to remember about exercise are that:

- The form of exercise should be enjoyable and not a task.
- You should be puffing at the end but not exhausted.
- To achieve aerobic effects you need to exercise at least three times a week for not less than 20 minutes each time, getting the pulse rate above the important lower index number without stress, while keeping it below the higher number to avoid cardiac strain.
- You should *never* hold your breath when exercising – keep your breathing regular, use your diaphragm, and breathe in and out through your mouth if this is more comfortable.

WATER EXERCISES

You can do more things in water than out of it, especially if your joints are stiff and aching, because water supports the body more than air does. Obviously a pool is going to provide greater scope than a bath, but you can still achieve a lot in a confined space. Any exercise (in or out of water) should be painless and should be performed slowly and deliberately. If you are standing in the bath or shower have a slip mat in place. Make sure that the water is warm and the room draught-free.

Basic Exercises for the Bath

These exercises are good for stiff or painful joints and muscles. Whatever part is stiff, restricted or uncomfortable should be allowed a few minutes of gentle soaking. Ideally the bath should have some Epsom salts and/or sea salt in it.

Gently move the part (knee, ankle, elbow, neck, or even back) in various directions, carefully paying attention to the direction(s) of maximum 'bind' or restriction, or which hurt, and the direction(s) of maximum ease where the part, or you, feels most comfortable. Then try one of the following three exercises. If the first or the second is successful, repeat it the next time you bathe. If it isn't, use the other exercise next time.

Exercise 1

This is most suitable for stiff and restricted parts that are not particularly painful.

Move the joint towards the most restricted position but not to the point of pain. Stay in this position for about 15 seconds and then see whether you can *without force or pain* go a little further towards the restricted direction. If you are successful, repeat until no further gain is possible, and stay there for about a minute before slowly returning to the starting position.

Exercise 2

This is most suitable for areas that are restricted and painful on movement, or just painful.

Take the joint towards the direction of maximum ease, where it feels to be most 'free' and unrestricted (take a minute or two to find this position). Hold this for a full minute and then gently see whether you can take it more easily in the previously restricted or painful direction.

Exercise 3

Slowly and deliberately move the joint as far as possible, while it is underwater, in all the directions that are *not* restricted or painful. Keep moving and repeat the directions that are 'easy', avoiding all painful movements. Do this for two or three minutes before resting. See how the area feels the next day. If it is easier, use this method again.

Aquarobics – Active Water Exercises

To achieve useful levels of toning exercise in water you need access to a swimming pool or the sea. As with all aerobic exercise, always stretch beforehand to 'warm up' the muscles in preparation for what is to come and to avoid injury. Get a book on warm-up exercises and do what is appropriate for your needs.

To achieve real toning benefit from water exercise join a class – there is no substitute for following an expert's lead.

Swimming – and Your Neck

If you want to go it alone in a pool then settle for swimming, or get hold of one of the many books now available on pool exercises. If you choose swimming, start with a few lengths or breadths of the pool and gradually train yourself to do as many as you can, using the pulse test to make sure that you are not overdoing it and that you are doing enough to make a difference to your fitness level.

Whether you are doing crawl or breast stroke, swimming places a lot of stress on your neck unless your face is in the water. You might want to avoid this strain by getting swimming goggles or a watertight face-mask and a snorkel, and swim face down in the water, breathing through the snorkel, raising your eyes just enough to see where you are going every now and then.

CAUTION: Stop whatever exercise you are doing if you:

- Feel tightness or pain in your chest
- Become severely breathless
- Become light-headed or dizzy or feel nausea
- Feel exhausted
- Lose muscle control

Stop and rest, and if the symptom persists call a doctor.

RECOGNIZING STRESS

You can easily recognize high stress levels when you show any of the following signs:

- Being more restless or easily upset than usual
- Difficulty in relaxing

- Disturbed sleep pattern
- Sighing a lot, or breathing less deeply than usual
- Difficulty in concentrating
- Feeling on edge
- An almost constant sense of anxiety

So what is to be done if you are feeling the effects of too much stress? Part of the answer is to learn to reduce your anxiety level, which may be a lot easier than you expect. You can work towards this in a number of different ways.

How Stressed Are You?

If you are currently stressed and not coping well with it you will answer YES to most of the following:

1. In stressful situations do you become edgy and nervous?

2. If you are in a stressful situation do you commonly get breathless, tight-chested and find yourself sighing and periodically taking deep breaths?

3. When upset or angry do you go bright red in the face?

4. If you had to speak to a group or meet new people would you feel physically sick, vomit or have diarrhoea?

5. If you are waiting to meet someone, or are feeling apprehensive about something, do you sweat, get strange feelings in the stomach and/or get goose-pimples on the skin?

6. In the same situation as question 5 does your pulse start to race or do you feel a pounding in the head?

7. If a sudden sound is heard do you get very startled and feel upset?

8. Do you grind your teeth and/or find yourself fiddling with your hands or fingers a lot?

The more YES answers to these questions, the more stress is affecting you right now, and the more you need to learn to relax and let go.

People who cope best with stress of any sort possess certain characteristics. If you already have most of these your need to do something about increasing your 'stress-proofing' will be far less important than if you lack the characteristics of good stress copers. The chances are that the more YES answers you gave to the questions above, the more 'a' answers you will give to the next four questions.

Do you:
a) dread change and feel threatened by it, or
b) welcome change as a challenge, an opportunity for development?

Do you:
a) find it difficult to get involved in discussion or socializing when you are in a room full of strangers, or
b) find yourself chatting comfortably and interacting with strangers?

Do you:
a) feel that 'things' happen to you and your family which you cannot control or deal with, or
b) that life-events are at least partially within your control and/or that you can deal with events when they occur.

Do you
a) feel that life in general moulds you and that what happens in your life is determined by fate, or
b) that you can influence and have some control over your own destiny?

The more 'b' answers the better; the more 'a' answers the more work there is for you to do in learning to take charge of your life. Starting to use hydrotherapy at home, where you are actually taking responsibility for your health and fitness, is an excellent way to begin this process.

If you have a cluster of 'a' answers there is likely also to be a tendency towards frequent feelings of anxiety and nervousness, a sense of failure, poor self esteem, lack of confidence, difficulty in concentrating or making decisions or easily expressing deeper feelings, and a tendency towards dwelling on either past or future events rather than on the present time.

As you practise deeper relaxation, improved breathing and improved dietary patterns, along with appropriate hydrotherapy measures, so you should become less anxious and self-critical and more self-confident, focused and decisive. Consider seeking professional counselling if there are major anxieties that remain unexpressed and unresolved.

Calming the Mind

The ripple effect of anything positive or negative in our emotions reaches into how energetic or lethargic you feel, how enthusiastic or listless you are, how vital or empty you seem to others. And it shows – in body language and in appearance.

The difference between being bright-eyed, alert, purposeful and ready for action, and being dull, droopy, unresponsive and unenthusiastic about anything and everything, can lie in as simple a factor as how well or badly you handle stress. The secret of coping with stress lies both in avoiding as much of it as you can, learning to cope with what cannot be avoided, and also learning to give your mind and body escape routes to relaxation in which balance can be restored.

There are a number of easily learned techniques which can help enormously in this direction, and any health-enhancing strategy needs to include them. The various hydrotherapy measures already described – constitutional hydrotherapy, various essential oil baths, neutral baths and the full sheet pack – combined with the use of essential oils and herbal infusions, the receiving of massage, regular pleasant forms of exercise and balanced nutrition all offer protection against the effects of stress. But they demand that one more ingredient be dealt with – your mind.

Muscular release

It is important to find a way to release tension from your muscles. This might call for massage, self-applied stretching (as in yoga), exercise, water therapy or better nutrition. Muscular release is the first step towards calming the mind, because the mind cannot be calm if your muscles are tense. Being relaxed also saves energy.

Diet

If you are to be really relaxed and able to cope with stress your diet should be nourishing, while your intake of 'tasty toxins' and stimulants should be as low as possible. Refer to the section on detox strategies

Full breathing

Your breathing should be full and free. This can be helped by massage, exercise, stretching, water therapy along with essential oils, and through the breathing exercise described below. Full breathing leads to better circulation and oxygenation and has specific effects on feelings of anxiety and being 'stressed out', since the body cannot relax or cope well with stress if it is poorly supplied with vital oxygen and nutrients.

Stress-Reducing Breathing Technique

There are many exercises to help improve breathing, but there is just one that has been shown in medical studies to be effective in reducing anxiety levels. This is an exercise based on traditional yogic breathing.

Place yourself in a comfortable (ideally seated/reclining) position, exhale slowly and *fully* through your partially open mouth, lips just barely separated. This out-breath should be performed slowly. Imagine that there is a candle flame about 6in (15cm) from your mouth and exhale, blowing out a thin stream of air in such a way as to *not* blow this out. As you exhale count silently to yourself to establish the length of the out-breath. An effective method for counting one second at a time is to say (silently) 'one hundred, two hundred, three hundred' and so on.

When you have exhaled fully, without causing any sense of strain in any way, allow the inhalation (through the nose) which follows to be full, free and uncontrolled. The complete exhalation which preceded the inhalation will have created a 'coiled spring' which you do not have to control in order to inhale. Once again count to yourself to establish how long your in-breath lasts. The counting is necessary because the timing of the inhalation and exhalation phases is a major feature of this exercise.

Without pausing to hold the breath exhale *fully and slowly*, through the mouth, blowing the air in a thin stream (again you should count to yourself at the same speed). Continue to repeat the inhalation and the exhalation for not less than 30 complete cycles.

The objective is that in time (some weeks of practising this twice daily – on waking and again later in the day) you should achieve an inhalation phase which lasts for two to three seconds, while the exhalation phase lasts from six to seven seconds – without any strain at all. Most importantly the exhalation should be slow and continuous. It is no use breathing the air out in two seconds and then simply waiting until the count reaches six, seven or eight before inhaling again.

By the time you have completed fifteen or so cycles any sense of anxiety which you previously felt should be much reduced, and if pain is a problem this should also have lessened.

Apart from *always* practising this once or twice daily, it is useful to repeat the exercise for a few minutes (about five cycles of inhalation/exhalation takes a minute) every hour if you are anxious, or whenever stress seem to be increasing. At the very least it should be practised on waking, and before bedtime, and if at all possible before meals

A Calm Mind

Once you have achieved relatively relaxed muscles and have learned full breathing, you need to learn to still and focus your mind, so releasing yourself from the constant internal chatter of daily events and anxieties. This can be achieved by regularly using a form of meditation which suits you. Meditation leads to a profound sense of being centred and at ease, which is apparent to those around you as your ability to concentrate and remember details is boosted and your whole being reflects calmness.

Relaxation technique (modified autogenic training)

There are a vast number of relaxation exercises, but one in particular seems to suit most people – try it and see. It needs repeating daily for a week or more before you can judge whether it is right for your personal needs. If other forms of relaxation suit you better, use them, since anything that produces a reduction of muscular tension and anxiety is going to give you more energy and help you feel and look better. Autogenic training is best learned from a fully trained instructor, but the following modified form is an excellent way of starting to learn to relax.

Lie on the floor or bed in a comfortable position, perhaps with

111

a small cushion under your head, knees bent if that makes your back feel easier, and with your eyes closed. Focus your attention on your right hand or arm and silently say to yourself, 'My right arm or hand feels heavy'. Try to see the arm relaxed and heavy, its weight sinking into the surface it is resting on. Feel its weight. Over a period of about a minute repeat the statement several times, and try to stay focused on the weight and heaviness of your hand or arm. You will almost certainly lose focus as your attention wanders from time to time. Staying focused is part of the training in the exercise, so don't feel angry, just go back to the arm and its heaviness. You may or may not be able to sense the heaviness – it doesn't matter too much at first. If you do, stay with it and enjoy the sense of release, of letting go, that comes with it.

Next, focus on your left hand or arm and do exactly the same thing for about a minute. Move to the left leg and then the right leg, giving each the same message that you gave to your arms.

Go back to your right hand or arm and silently say, 'My right arm is feeling warm (or hot)'. After a minute or so go to the left hand or arm, the left leg and then finally the right leg, each time with the warming message. If warmth is sensed stay with it for a while and feel it spread. Enjoy it. Again, try to keep your attention focused.

Finally, focus on your forehead and affirm that it feels cool and refreshed. Stay with this for a minute before completing the exercise. By repeating the whole exercise at least once a day (10 to 15 minutes is all it will take) you will gradually find you can stay focused on each region and sensation (warmth, heaviness, coolness) for the full minute in each case. 'Heaviness' represents what you feel when muscles relax and 'warmth' is what you feel when your circulation to an area is increased, while 'coolness' is the opposite, a reduction in circulation for a short while.

You can use the new skills you have gained to focus on any area where you wish to create a positive change in your health. For example, 'I am calm and relaxed', 'My aching back is easing and relaxing', 'I feel full of energy', 'My skin is clear' and so on. When you are internally verbalizing this sort of message you are in fact practising visualization, especially if you can stay focused on the message and area and if you repeat the message frequently, several times a day.

Creative visualization

And finally, once you have taken care of muscular tension and breathing, and your mind is still, you need to exercise it in creative visualization and guided imagery – creating pictures in your mind – to round out your personal journey towards health and happiness. Depending on your belief system this can include spiritual dimensions and should certainly allow for growth in your personal sense of worth and usefulness.

To be most effective, visualization should follow on from deep relaxation. Positive visualization means using 'mental pictures', creating harmonious, uplifting and safe images – a flowery sunlit meadow by a sparkling river; a quiet beach scene; a favourite garden or room – to produce a profound state of contentment. You simply see such a scene in your mind's eye, and then imagine yourself there. The next stage is to employ your mind to encourage any particular health-enhancing state (peaceful tranquillity, energized well-being, relaxation, strength, and so on) you wish to develop and enhance.

Whatever visualization image you construct it is absolutely essential that relaxation be achieved first. Visualization adds just one more dimension to relaxation, allowing the mind to become involved more actively in achieving health gains.

As indicated in previous chapters, a great deal of hydrotherapy can be self-applied, and this is often what chiropractors, osteopaths and naturopaths will recommend. Some forms of hydrotherapy, however, are specialized and need expert application. If you want to find a practitioner using hydrotherapy, or wish to study aspects of this fascinating branch of healing, the contact details and books listed on the following pages offer a useful starting point.

CONCLUSION

What emerges from a review of ancient and modern hydrotherapy is a clear message – water therapy can help to heal you, and it can help to keep you healthy. Hydrotherapy can, should be and often is integrated with almost all other forms of health promotion, since no more simple and efficient approach exists to help circulation, ease pain, reduce fatigue, clear congestion, induce calm, boost immune function, improve skin tone and function, or simply to enhance beauty and wellbeing. The variety of useful ways in which water can be used in health promotion; its unique physical and chemical characteristics (whether as ice, as water alone, or containing other substances, or as steam); its easy availability; its low cost – all add up to a powerful validation of hydrotherapy as a self-help approach which should be used in every home.

Notes

Chapter 1

[1] *Physiotherapy*, vol 76, no 4, pp 207–10, April 1990

Chapter 4

[1] *Journal of the Royal Society of Medicine*, vol 80, pp 776–7, December 1987
[2] Sutherland, A, *An Attempt to Ascertain the Virtues of Bath and Bristol Waters*, Frederick and Leake, pp 352–3, London 1764
[3] *British Medical Journal*, vol 291, pp 1747–51, 21–28 December 1985
[4] Jensen, Dr Steen, 'Treatment of first episode acute anal fissure', *British Medical Journal*, vol 292, 3 May 1986

Chapter 5

[1] Standish, L, 'One year open trial of naturopathic treatment of HIV infection', *Journal of Naturopathic Medicine* 3(1), pp 42–64, 1992
Martin, L, *et al*, 'Disinfection and inactivation of human T-lymphotrophic virus-111 lymphadenopathy-associated virus', *Journal of Infectious Disease*, 152(2), pp 300–403, 1985
Weatherburn, H, 'Hyperthermia and Aids Treatment', *British Journal of Radiology*, 61, pp 862–3, 1989

Temperature Conversion

F°	C°	F°	C°	F°	C°	F°	C°
32	0.0	50	10.0	68	20.0	86	30.0
33	0.6	51	10.6	69	20.6	87	30.6
34	1.1	52	11.1	70	21.1	88	31.1
35	1.7	53	11.7	71	21.7	89	31.7
36	2.2	54	12.2	72	22.2	90	32.2
37	2.8	55	12.8	73	22.8	91	32.8
38	3.3	56	13.3	74	23.3	92	33.3
39	3.9	57	13.9	75	23.9	93	33.9
40	4.4	58	14.4	76	24.4	94	34.4
41	5.0	59	15.0	77	25.0	95	35.0
42	5.6	60	15.6	78	25.6	96	35.6
43	6.1	61	16.1	79	26.1	97	36.1
44	6.7	62	16.7	80	26.7	98	36.7
45	7.2	63	17.2	81	27.2	99	37.2
46	7.8	64	17.8	82	27.8	100	37.8
47	8.3	65	18.3	83	28.3		
48	8.9	66	18.9	84	28.9		
49	9.4	67	19.4	85	29.4		

Further Reading

Alexander, Jane, *Supertherapies*, Bantam Books, London, 1996.

Boyle, Wade, and Saine, Andre, *Naturopathic Hydrotherapy*, Buckeye Naturopathic Press, East Palastine, Ohio, 1988

Buchma, D, *The Complete Book of Water Therapy*, New York, 1979

Kellogg, J H, *Rational Hydrotherapy*, F A Davis Co, Philadelphia, 1903

Kirchfeld, Friedhelm, and Boyle, Wade, *Nature Doctors*, Medicina Biologica, Portland, Oregon, 1994

Kneipp, Sebastian, *My Water Cure*, William Blackwood & Sons, London, 1893

Licht, Sidney, *Medical Hydrology*, Elizabeth Licht, New Haven, Connecticut, 1963

Lindlahr, Henry, *Natural Therapeutics Practice*, C W Daniel Co, Saffron Walden, 1981

Useful Addresses

Australia

Australian Natural Therapists Association
PO Box 856
Caloundra QLD 4551
Tel.: +1800 817 577
E-mail: anta1 955@bigpond.com
Website: http://www.anta.com.au/

Canada

Canadian College of Naturopathic Medicine
Tel.: 416 498 1255
E-mail: info@ccnm.edu
Website: http://www.ccnm.edu/

UK

British College of Naturopathy and Osteopathy
Lief House
120–122 Finchley Road
London NW3 5HR
Tel.: 020 7435 6464
Fax: 020 7431 3630
Website: http://www.bcno.org.uk/

Tyringham Naturopathic Clinic
Park Farm
Newport Pagnell,
Buckinghamshire MK16 8LG
Tel.: 01908 551 935
Fax: 01908 551450
E-mail: info@tyringhamclinic@co.uk
Website: http://www.tyringhamclinic.co.uk

USA

The American Association of Naturopathic Physicians
8201 Greensboro Drive, Suite 300
McLean, VA 22102
Tel.: 703 610 9037
Tel. (Toll-Free): 877 969 2267
Website: http://www.naturopathic.org/

Bastyr University
14500 Juanita Dr. NE
Kenmore, WA 98028–4966
Tel.: 425 823 1300
Website: http://www.bastyr.edu/

National College of Naturopathic Medicine
Website: http://www.ncnm.edu/

Southwest College of Naturopathic Medicine
Website: http://www.scnm.edu/

Index

Index